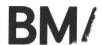

SIXTH EDITION

SILVER'S JOINT AND SOFT TISSUE INJECTION

INJECTING WITH CONFIDENCE

D1388762

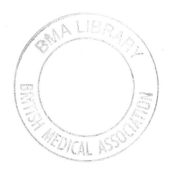
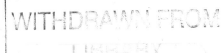

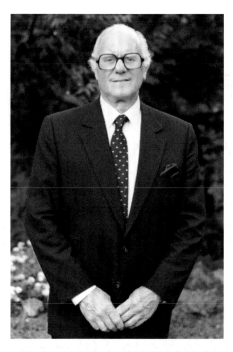

Trevor Silver (1927–2011)

Dr Silver was a general practitioner (GP) with an interest in the management of musculoskeletal conditions, notably injection therapy. Throughout his career, he was interested in education and training. For many years, he was Regional Adviser to South West Thames Region British Postgraduate Medical Federation and held a number of important roles within the Royal College of General Practitioners, including Chair and Provost of the South West Thames Faculty. He chaired many management, education and research committees, including the local division of the BMA and his regional health authority regional research committee.

He was a GP advisor to the Arthritis and Rheumatism Council and a trainer to the Royal Army Medical Corps (RAMC). He contributed to original research on the regional inequalities of GP training in inner city areas. He travelled widely to deliver his highly regarded soft tissue and joint injection workshops and published the successful book, *Joint and Soft Tissue Injection*. (Adapted from *BMJ* 2011; 343:d7233 with permission from BMJ Publishing Group Ltd.)

SIXTH EDITION

SILVER'S JOINT AND SOFT TISSUE INJECTION

INJECTING WITH CONFIDENCE

EDITED BY

DAVID SILVER FRCR FRCP

Consultant Musculoskeletal Radiologist
Royal Devon and Exeter NHS Foundation Trust
Past President, British Society of Skeletal Radiologists
UK

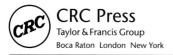

CRC Press
Taylor & Francis Group
Boca Raton London New York

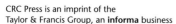

CRC Press is an imprint of the
Taylor & Francis Group, an **informa** business

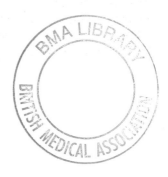

CRC Press
Taylor & Francis Group
6000 Broken Sound Parkway NW, Suite 300
Boca Raton, FL 33487-2742

© 2019 by Taylor & Francis Group, LLC
CRC Press is an imprint of Taylor & Francis Group, an Informa business

No claim to original U.S. Government works

Printed on acid-free paper

International Standard Book Number-13: 978-1-138-60417-9 (Paperback)
978-1-138-60420-9 (Hardback)

**Visit the Taylor & Francis Web site at
http://www.taylorandfrancis.com**

**and the CRC Press Web site at
http://www.crcpress.com**

Contents

Preface to the first edition

In this book the author has provided a concise desk-top guide that will provide the practitioner with a comprehensive description and illustration for treatment of most common joint and soft tissue disorders that can be treated effectively in general practice. Medical education workshops organised by tutors are a good introduction to the subject, and realistic models (simulators) may be used as teaching aids to allow repeated practice of all the techniques a practitioner could wish to learn, thus avoiding the necessity of learning and practicing on live patients. Models of the shoulder, wrist and hand, knee joint and elbow joint are available. These are marketed by Limbs and Things Ltd of Bristol and I acted as their consultant in the development of these models, which have proved invaluable in the teaching workshops.

Practitioners will gain much stimulation and satisfaction from treating patients with such a variety of soft tissue and joint conditions. Patients will benefit from receiving prompt and efficient therapy, thus avoiding the all too common problem within the National Health Service of long waiting lists for hospital appointments.

This book will reinforce the practice and teaching of injecting joints and soft tissue disorders or lesions, thus achieving the aim of imparting the ability to 'inject with confidence'.

Trevor Silver
January 1996

Preface to the second edition

I have conducted many practical skills workshops teaching joint and soft tissue injection techniques. More than 5000 doctors have attended these sessions conducted in the United Kingdom and throughout Europe, Asia and Africa. Interestingly, it is not just the minor surgery list in the NHS that has encouraged this increased learning activity, as family practitioners worldwide are becoming much more interested in developing their skills and providing expert joint injection services to their patients. This updated and revised edition includes most of the injection skills family practitioners would want to undertake in their daily practice, and provides most of the answers to questions raised by doctors wishing to provide this service to their patients.

Trevor Silver
September 1998

Preface to the third edition

This manual provides detailed instruction regarding steroid injection of joint and soft tissue lesions. The evidence base for these therapies is still sparse and has not advanced since the second edition was published. In spite of this, the consensus of opinion appears to support the value of this form of therapy and general practitioners, rheumatologists and orthopaedic surgeons continue to rely on these techniques and principles of therapy. Increasing numbers of GPs worldwide are attending lectures and practical skills workshops, either to learn or to refresh their knowledge of and skills in joint injection therapies.

This third edition benefits from an additional chapter by Dr David Silver, Consultant Radiologist, who has a special interest in musculoskeletal imaging. He elucidates the role of the hospital specialist in the further management of these disorders. Particular attention is paid to those patients who do not respond to initial injection therapy and where specialist referral may be advisable. The need for imaging, particularly the use of ultrasound, magnetic resonance imaging and image-guided intervention, is discussed.

It is my expectation that as this subject is practised by increasing numbers of practitioners, more evidence will be forthcoming. The need to agree criteria for diagnosis, techniques of injection and therapy will inevitably facilitate the organisation of more meaningful and informative studies.

More research is needed to establish a uniform method for defining these individual disorders and standardising injection techniques, as well as developing outcome measures that are valid, reliable and responsive in these study populations.

Trevor Silver
September 2001

Preface to the fourth edition

The fact that the publishers have requested a fourth edition of this book confirms that interest in injecting joints and soft tissues continues to flourish.

General practitioners and hospital doctors not only in the UK, but worldwide, are finding that these practical skills are rewarding in primary care as well as in hospital care. The fact that this book is now published in several languages confirms this interest.

Since writing the last edition there has been a noticeable increase in published work, trials and reviews of the literature on the whole range of treatments used in musculoskeletal conditions. Thus, the evidence base is now very comprehensive and a recent restricted Medline search produced over 3500 references. Consequently 'injecting with confidence' is not just a matter of learning about the presentation of the many conditions responding to this form of therapy. Rather, it is the added confidence produced by this evidence base that this subject is now accepted both clinically and therapeutically.

Viscosupplementation is increasingly used to treat a variety of joints with the added prospects of success and prolongation of pain relief. This edition includes recent references and I would encourage readers to read the relevant papers to broaden their horizons of knowledge and so expand their confidence in their management of these conditions.

The evidence for the success of teaching and practical skills workshops, recently published, further confirms my confidence that this subject is now on a much more substantial foundation educationally. It is rewarding to realise that my experience of the last 15 years or so in teaching this subject with practical skills workshops, using simulator models and lectures, has been rewarded by the increasing evidence of a larger number of doctors continuing to practise these skills.

Trevor Silver
February 2007

Preface to the fifth edition

The popularity of this book has been further enhanced by the increasing interest of professionals treating musculoskeletal disorders. Physiotherapists and sports medicine specialists and podiatrists are increasingly combining steroid injections with physiotherapeutic measures of treatment. Because of this, it is necessary that information is available to all practitioners so that a comprehensive approach to successful therapy is achieved.

I am delighted to welcome David MacLellan as a contributing author. His contribution as a sports medicine specialist and physiotherapist complements this book.

General practitioners worldwide are increasingly injecting corticosteroids and this book contributes to their education, as well as their continuing need to attend practical skills workshops and courses.

This edition has further included sections on the elbow joint and iliotibial band syndrome. Further updating on the concepts of greater trochanter pain syndrome is included.

Our aim is to ensure that all therapists have a comprehensive and clear handbook that ensures a high standard of success in treating these conditions.

The increase, worldwide, of physical exercise and recreation as the key to good health and longevity makes this book an essential tool towards the education of the many general practitioners, physiotherapists, orthopaedic physicians, surgeons, podiatrists and radiologists. It is interesting that so many disciplines are increasingly engaging in treating these musculoskeletal disorders.

Trevor Silver
October 2010

Preface to the sixth edition

I was asked to write a chapter on Image Guided Injections by my Father for the third edition of this text, and subsequently Trevor Silver went on to edit two further editions with valuable updates. The last edition was produced as the realisation of a lifetime ambition, at a time when my Father was terminally ill; he strived to complete the text as he never could give up his drive for educational excellence.

It is my privilege to edit the sixth edition of this valuable book, which has been acknowledged as a desktop guide to injection therapy and published in five languages. This new edition has built on the key messages in the previous editions and includes new chapters that will help the practitioner undertaking injections.

The focus has been to include information that furthers knowledge and addresses diagnosis of early inflammatory arthritis, evidence base for steroid injections and specific guidance on best physiotherapy management to supplement injections of soft tissue disorders. This edition has been revised to include best evidence-based information and address important issues around patient safety, including consent for injections.

I am very grateful for contributions from Dr Bashaar Boyce, Consultant Rheumatologist, Dr Ravik Mascarenhas, Consultant Rheumatologist, Dr Anish Patel, Consultant Musculoskeletal Radiologist, and Alison Smeatham, Extended Scope Physiotherapist, who have kindly contributed the relevant chapters.

The key messages are preserved in this edition, as Trevor Silver's original text has been the basis for many practitioners gaining the skill and confidence to treat patients using injection therapy. His legacy continues in this updated version, reviewed to address current developments and current changes to medical practice in line with current guidance.

Trevor Silver would be proud to know that his lifetime of experience in treatment of soft tissue disorders has continued to expand in knowledge and evidence, and I hope the readers will benefit accordingly.

David Silver
October 2018

Introduction

INJECTING WITH CONFIDENCE

The development of relatively insoluble corticosteroids has provided doctors with a most useful and effective treatment for the painful musculoskeletal conditons that commonly occur in soft tissues and inflammatory arthropathies. Corticosteroids are potent anti-inflammatory and anti-allergic compounds presented in injectable form in sterile-packed ampoules and vials.

Patients present to their general practitioners (GPs) as a first contact, complaining of pain caused by soft tissue conditions affecting tendons, tendon sheaths or musculotendinous junctions, or of painful joints themselves. The cause of these problems is often repetitive strain of a tendon, sport, occupationally induced or a part of a degenerative process resulting in tenderness and pain on movement of the affected structure. Although many of these conditions may be self-limiting, effective treatment using steroid injections as part of the treatment is often dramatic and, when accurately diagnosed and accurately injected, produces relief in most cases, allowing effective mobilisation and physiotherapy to have an opportunity for maximum benefit.

Both hospital doctors and GPs are ideally placed to treat these disorders, and as most of these patients present in the primary care setting, these problems, quite properly, are considered to be an important part of the general practice curriculum.

Knowledge of the functional (clinical) anatomy, together with learning each individual skill or technique of injection, leads to confidence in treating all these disorders, and it is the aim of this book to provide a comprehensive knowledge and demonstration of skills in an illustrative way, thus imparting to every practitioner the ability to 'inject with confidence'. Making an accurate anatomical and pathological diagnosis implies a specific indication for steroid injection, thus assuring the patient prompt relief. There is no place nowadays for treatment by trial and error. For example, the practice of seeing a patient with shoulder pain and injecting steroid before making a diagnosis, arranging then to review in 1 to 2 weeks' time in the hope of providing relief, is not acceptable. Rather, the doctor should always be in the position of reassuring the patient of prompt relief of pain and of having made an accurate diagnosis before giving treatment.

Practitioners will complement injection therapy as appropriate with analgesic drugs and physiotherapy. They will also be able to advise rest of the affected part for 24–48 hours after the injection, if appropriate, and suitable mobilisation thereafter, leading to a resumption of full activity.

About the author

Dr David Silver studied Medicine at St Bartholomew's Hospital, London, and after gaining MRCP trained in Radiology at University Hospitals Bristol NHS Foundation Trust, Bristol, before undertaking a Fellowship at the Princess Alexandra Hospital, Brisbane, Australia. He has been a Consultant at the Royal Devon and Exeter NHS Foundation Trust, Exeter, since 1997 and has established a comprehensive musculoskeletal (MSK) diagnostic and interventional service in association with the renowned Princess Elizabeth Orthopaedic Centre, being one of the first NHS Trusts to introduce MSK ultrasound and guided injections.

He developed one of the first NHS centres for shockwave therapy and has been a Specialist Adviser to the National Institute for Health and Care Excellence for over 12 years.

Dr Silver is currently the President of the British Society of Skeletal Radiologists, has advised the Department of Health on imaging issues, including the 18 week referral to treatment (RTT) pathway, and been a member of the National Imaging Board.

He was a member of the Imaging Committee for the 2012 Olympic Games and was a volunteer at the games, providing MSK imaging and intervention. He has provided specialist imaging and interventional advice for Exeter City Football Club and Somerset Cricket Club for many years.

Contributors

Bashaar Boyce MBChB, BSc, MRCP
Consultant Rheumatologist
Royal National Hospital for Rheumatic Diseases
Bath, England

Ravik Mascarenhas BMedSci, BMBS, MRCP
Consultant Rheumatologist
Royal Devon and Exeter Foundation Trust
Exeter, England

Anish Patel FRCR
Consultant Radiologist
Royal Orthopaedic Hospital
Birmingham, England

David Silver FRCR, FRCP
Consultant Musculoskeletal Radiologist
President British Society of Skeletal Radiologists
Royal Devon and Exeter NHS Foundation Trust
Exeter, England

Alison Smeatham MSc., MCSP, FSOM
Extended Scope Physiotherapist
Royal Devon and Exeter NHS Foundation Trust
Exeter, England

Dr Anish Patel contributed Chapter 2, Dr Bashaar Boyce and Dr Ravik Mascarenhas contributed Chapter 4, and Ms Alison Smeatham contributed the Physiotherapy sections in Chapters 5–10.

Abbreviations

anti-CCP	anti-citrullinated c-peptide
BMI	body mass index
DAS	disease activity score
DLCO	low total diffusion capacity
DMARD	disease-modifying antirheumatic drug
ESWL	extracorporeal shockwave lithotripsy
ESWT	extracorporeal shockwave therapy
GP	general practitioner
GTPS	greater trochanter pain syndrome
INR	international normalised ratio
MMPI	Minnesota Multiphasic Personality Inventory
MRI	magnetic resonance imaging
NHS	National Health Service
NICE	National Institute for Health and Care Excellence
NOACs	novel oral anticoagulants
NSAID	non-steroidal anti-inflammatory drug
POLICE	protection, optimal loading, ice, compression and elevation
QOL	quality of life
RA	rheumatoid arthritis
RCT	randomised controlled trial
RF	rheumatoid factor
RICE	rest, ice, compression and elevation
VAS	visual analogue scale

CHAPTER 1

Incidence and general principles

There are over eight million people in the UK who are suffering from some form of rheumatic disease, and it has been estimated that about one-fifth of all general practitioner (GP) consultations may be attributed to some form of rheumatological or musculoskeletal problem.

Shoulder complaints account for one in every 170 adult patient consultations per year, whereas back problems may account for one in 30 adult patient consultations annually. Thus, it is apparent that back problems are approximately five times more common in practice than are shoulder problems.[1] Even so, GPs may well expect to see 20–30 shoulder problems a year in a practice of average list size. Billings and Mole recorded in a prospective study in a London general practice that 10.6% of patients presented with a new rheumatological problem.[2] Of these, 30% were lumbosacral problems, 15% cervical spine problems, 26% degenerative joint disease and 20% soft tissue non-articular rheumatism. Trauma, including sports injuries, accounted for 35% of these problems. The incidence in English and Dutch general practice has been estimated at 6.6–25 per 1000 registered patients per year.[3] The lower annual reported incidence occurred in England and Wales and the higher figure in The Netherlands. In assessing the frequency of the cause of shoulder pain, glenohumeral instability is more likely in under-25 year olds, tendinosis ('impingement') in the 25–40-year-old age group and frozen shoulder (adhesive capsulitis) in the over-40-year-old age group, with a higher incidence in individuals with diabetes. The term 'impingement' means that the inflamed supraspinatus tendon impinges under the acromion process. Inflammatory joint disease accounts for about 5.5% of these problems, and there is often a case for injecting an inflamed joint with steroid, providing a clinical diagnosis of the type of arthritis has been confirmed beforehand.

It is therefore immediately apparent that GPs are well placed to diagnose and effectively treat all these disorders in their own surgeries, if for no other reason than that the patient will then be assured of prompt and effective treatment for what is often a painful and disabling condition, thus eliminating the frequent long delay many patients experience in obtaining hospital outpatient clinic appointments.

Confirming a diagnosis of these conditions involves examining the active, passive and resisted movements of muscles and affected joints, and relating these to the clinical anatomy. Where there is doubt, radiographs, blood investigations, including erythrocyte sedimentation rate, magnetic resonance imaging (MRI) and ultrasound scans, may all be helpful in differential diagnosis. A careful history, including the onset of pain, trauma, occupational hazards, sports, gardening and housework, is essential. This careful assessment will give the practitioner confidence in managing these conditions accurately and successfully.

As with everything in medicine, it is always wise to take a very careful and complete history; so often the clinician makes a diagnosis before even examining the patient. For example, it is well known that tendon rupture may be hereditary, and a careful history may well reveal that a patient with an Achilles or a long head of biceps tendon problem also had a mother or grandmother with a similar problem. Naturally, this would alert one to the fact that it would be unwise to inject steroid around that tendon. Steroids are harmful substances when used inappropriately and, in the present climate of litigation, should never be injected into the substance of a tendon. A patient suffering a tendon rupture who has had a steroid injection in the 1 to 2 weeks beforehand would all too often be advised that this was because he or she had received a steroid injection. In actual fact, the situation would be likely to have been related to the hereditary nature of the condition. It is wise to make an accurate anatomical diagnosis on each patient by careful examination and demonstration of the functional anatomy. This is particularly important when diagnosing the cause of shoulder pain. A good understanding of the anatomy of the shoulder joint, its capsule and the rotator cuff will enable a diagnosis of the condition that the doctor knows will specifically respond to treatment with a steroid injection. This applies to all the conditions that may so easily be treated in the GP surgery, and these will be described in detail in the following chapters.

An aseptic technique should be used for every injection. Steroids are potent anti-inflammatories and in the presence of infection can spell disaster. Consequently, in the presence of local sepsis, such as cellulitis, furunculosis or other staphylococcal infection, introducing a steroid by injection should be avoided. Similarly, any suspicion of sepsis in the joint is an absolute contraindication to injecting steroids. In the presence of systemic infections, one must also exercise caution when using steroids. In the early days when tuberculosis was prevalent, clinicians exercised great caution and avoided the use of steroid medication for fear of exacerbating the illness, and this warning must still be valid today. In fact, in some areas, an increased incidence of tuberculosis is again evident, and vigilance is advised.

Defence organisations advise their members to wear sterile gloves when undertaking minor surgery procedures, including joint injections. Always be seen washing the hands beforehand and, where possible, use a 'no-touch' aseptic technique. Always use single-dose vials or ampoules, where possible, to avoid introducing contaminants into the injection solutions.

Sterilise the injection area and the vial cap using appropriate sterilisation technique according to local practice and best practice. This allows the operator to swab liberally and ensures safe working conditions. Nowadays, most doctors have ready access to gamma-irradiated sterile syringes and needles, which may only be used once and then safely disposed of. Inject carefully and unhurriedly. This is mentioned deliberately in order to underline that the patient may often be apprehensive before what is reputedly a painful injection. It is necessary to cast an appearance of calm in the operator and so help towards making the patient more relaxed. A relaxed patient will have more relaxed muscles, thus ensuring that the injection allows the solution to simply glide in, making the whole procedure easy and requiring no visible force on the syringe plunger. In fact, with all these injections, the agent should be felt to glide in easily and require the minimum of force to introduce. As in all procedures, there is the exception, and it must be stated that when injecting the denser fibrous tissues of musculotendinous junctions, as with tennis and golfer's elbow (lateral and medial epicondylitis), there may well be some resistance to the injection; in these cases, it is wise to ensure that the needle is firmly secured to the syringe.

FREQUENCY OF INJECTION

There is no firm rule regarding how frequently one may inject one symptomatic joint or soft tissue area, or one person, with several co-existent diagnoses. Generally, one must assume that the lowest number of injections and the lowest dose practicable should be employed. Although intra-articular steroid preparations are not likely to be systemically absorbed, some absorption will inevitably take place.

Consequently, the more frequently injections are given, the greater the likelihood, hypothetically, that the patient may exhibit all the unattractive qualities of long-term steroid administration, and we are all aware of the undesirable effects that this produces. One only needs to remember the patients who, in the past, were prescribed long-term steroids for asthma or rheumatoid arthritis to recall the possible side effects.

The general advice usually proffered is that, where necessary, one may inject a steroid at no more than 3- to 4-weekly intervals, and probably no more than three or four times into one lesion in the course of any one year. The author's view is that if two or three injections have not produced the desired and expected benefit, one should review the diagnosis. Certainly, if additional steroid medication is given, one should expect the patient to experience the undesirable effects associated with prolonged steroid medication.

This raises the question of why an injection may not produce the expected outcome. This should be a consideration after the first non-successful attempt, and the clinician should reconsider if they have made the correct diagnosis or targeted the correct location. It is worthwhile to consider an image-guided injection in these circumstances.

ANTICOAGULATION

The decision to undertake injections in patients on anticoagulants must be carefully assessed.

Current practice and evidence would suggest that stopping anticoagulation medication is not indicated as long as the international normalised ratio (INR) is within therapeutic range and does not exceed 4.5.

The risk of cessation of anticoagulation medication may outweigh the benefits of injection, so every patient must be assessed on an individual basis by the clinician.

Patients who are taking novel oral anticoagulants (NOACs) may also not need to stop treatment. Manufacturers produce specific advice, which should be heeded.[4-6]

CHOICE OF STEROID

There are many steroid preparations on the market for intra-articular and soft tissue use. They are relatively insoluble, consequently exerting a longer-lasting local effect, and are not absorbed systemically to any great degree. They should be injected into the substance of the lesion, the tender spot or the joint space. In some lesions, it is advisable to mix the steroid beforehand with local anaesthetic, whereas, in others such mixing will not take place; this will be discussed when describing each individual technique. Some preparations are marketed with steroid and local anaesthetic pre-mixed. This has the disadvantage of not allowing the operator the flexibility of titrating the preferred amounts or doses of local anaesthetic or steroid for each particular injection. This may be quite important when, for example, treating a painful recurrent condition, such as plantar fasciitis, and the requirement for local anaesthetic may vary in type and quantity (*see* following page).

Three commonly-used preparations are:

- Methylprednisolone acetate 40 mg/ml (Depo-Medrone®).
- Triamcinolone hexacetonide 20 mg/ml (Aristospan®).
- Triamcinolone acetonide 40 mg/ml (Kenalog®).

These preparations increase in potency and length of action in the order of the list, and, conversely, they decrease in volume for dose in that order. In effect, this means that triamcinolone acetonide will produce a longer-lasting effect in a comparatively smaller volume dose. This effect is clinically beneficial if one recalls that some of these injections, for example, those into dense tissue such as the tenoperiosteal junction in tennis elbow, can be quite painful. Therefore, the smaller the injection volume the better, to decrease the pain of the injection while at the same time delivering a very effective dose of steroid.

There are some occasions on which one will wish to mix the steroid with local anaesthetic, and others when it is inadvisable to add local anaesthetic; these will be discussed in the ensuing technique descriptions. Both hydrocortisone acetate and triamcinolone acetonide have product licences allowing one to pre-mix with lidocaine or bupivacaine. Methylprednisolone does not have such a licence, but the manufacturer of Depo-Medrone® produces a ready-mixed preparation with lidocaine 10 mg/ml.

CONTRAINDICATIONS TO THE USE OF STEROIDS

Active tuberculosis, ocular herpes and acute psychosis are considered to be absolute contraindications to glucocorticoid therapy, although the minimal systemic activity after local injection may permit its cautious use. Never inject steroids into infected joints. Where there is any suspicion, always aspirate any effusion and send it to the laboratory for culture of microorganisms before considering injecting. Similarly, diabetes, hypertension, osteoporosis and hyperthyroidism are listed as possible contraindications. Do not inject steroid into a joint with a prosthesis. Hypersensitivity to one of the ingredients of the injection is a definite contraindication. In pregnancy, one should take care; corticosteroids are certainly contraindicated in the first 16 weeks of pregnancy. It may be a fine clinical judgement of whether or not to use steroids, for example, in carpal tunnel syndrome, which is a common condition in middle pregnancy; caution must undoubtedly be exercised. It must also be remembered that prolonged or repeated use in weight-bearing joints may result in further degeneration. No more than two or three joints in a patient should be treated at the same time.

Never attempt to inject into the substance of a tendon, but always ensure that the steroid is injected into the space between the tendon and the tendon sheath in tenosynovitis.

LOCAL ANAESTHETIC

There are occasions in which one will wish to use local anaesthetic mixed with the steroid, and others when this is not advised. Lidocaine HCl 1% Plain is probably the most effective and commonly-used agent. This anaesthetic is extremely effective; its onset is immediate, and its effect will last for two to four hours. Where it is desirable to produce a longer-lasting local anaesthetic effect, for example, in the case of a recurrent plantar fasciitis, which is a very painful condition, it is sometimes useful to use bupivacaine plain 0.25% or 0.5% (Marcaine® Plain). The effect of this may last from 5 to 16 hours.

With both these local agents, it is undesirable and unnecessary to use adrenaline mixed with the anaesthetic solution.

There is evidence that Marcaine® may have a damaging effect on cartilage and, in some countries, it is no longer licenced for this indication.[7,8]

POST-INJECTION ADVICE

Following a steroid injection, the patient is advised to rest the joint or affected part for 2 or 3 days. This advice is not necessarily based on evidence, but may help patients improve without continued aggravation of their condition related to physical activity. Patients are advised not to carry heavy bags or shopping for a couple of days. Also the patient should not undertake any of the painful movements for a couple of days, after which a slow return to normal pain-free activity is permissible. Occasionally, the use of a sling following injection of a painful shoulder or tennis elbow is acceptable, but this should be discarded after the pain has resolved.

REFERENCES

1 Department of Health and Social Services (1986) *Morbidity Statistics from General Practice: The Third National Study (1981–1982)*. HMSO, London, UK.

2 Billings RA and Mole KF (1977) Rheumatology in general practice: a survey in world rheumatology year 1977. *J R Coll Gen Pract.* **27**: 721–725.

3 Croft P (1993) Soft tissue rheumatism. In: AJ Silman and MC Hochberg (Eds.) *Epidemiology of the Rheumatic Diseases.* Oxford Medical Publications, Oxford, UK.

4 Conway R, O'Shea FD, Cunnane G, Doran MF (2013) Safety of joint and soft tissue injections on warfarin anticoagulation. *Clin Rheumatol.* **32** (12): 1811–1814.

5 Ahmed I, Gertner E (2012) Safety of arthrocentesis and joint injection in patients receiving anticoagulation at therapeutic levels. *Am J Med.* **125** (3): 265–219.

6   Medical Information Updated 10 October 2013. *Boehringer Ingelheim.*

7   Webb ST and Ghosh S (2009) Intra-articular bupivacaine: potentially chondro-toxic? *Br J Anaesth.***102** (4): 439–441.

8   Chu CR *et al* (2010) In vivo effects of single intra-articular injection of 0.5% bupiva-caine on articular cartilage. *J Bone Joint Surg Am.* **92** (3): 599–608.

FURTHER READING

Aly AR *et al.* (2015) Ultrasound-guided shoulder girdle injections are more accurate and more effective than landmark-guided injections: a systematic review and meta-analysis. *Br J Sports Med.* **49** (16): 1042–1049.

Arroll B and Goodyear-Smith F (2005) Corticosteroid injections for painful shoulder: a meta-analysis. *Br J Gen Pract.* **55**: 224–228.

Bee WW and Thing J (2017) Ultrasound-guided injections in primary care: evidence, costs, and suggestions for change. *Br J Gen Pract.* **67** (661): 378–379.

Bell AD and Conaway D (2005) Corticosteroid injections for painful shoulders. *Int J Clin Pract.* **59**: 1178–1186.

Bloom JE *et al.* (2012) Image-guided versus blind glucocorticoid injection for shoulder pain. *Cochrane Database Syst Rev.* **15** (8): CD009147.

Chard M *et al* (1988) The long-term outcome of rotator cuff tendinosis: a review study. *Br J Rheumatol.* **27**: 385–389.

Cobley TDD *et al.* (2003) Ultrasound-guided steroid injection for osteoarthritis of the trapeziometacarpal joint of the thumb. *Eur J Plast Surg.* **26** (1): 47–49.

Cucurullo S *et al* (2004) Musculoskeletal injection skills competency: a method for development and assessment. *Am J Phys Med Rehabil.* **83** (6): 479–484.

D'Agostino MA and Schmidt WA (2013) Ultrasound-guided injections in rheumatology: actual knowledge on efficacy and procedures. *Best Pract Res Clin Rheumatol.* **27** (2): 283–294.

Daniels EW *et al.* (2018) Existing evidence on ultrasound-guided injections in sports medicine. *Orthop J Sports Med.* **6** (2): 2325967118756576.

Gallacher S *et al.* (2018) A randomized controlled trial of arthroscopic capsular release versus hydrodilatation in the treatment of primary frozen shoulder. *J Shoulder Elbow Surg.* **27** (8): 1401–1406.

Grahame R (2005) Efficacy of 'Hands On' soft tissue injection courses for general practitioners using live patients. *Poster Presentation at Rheumatology Conference.* Personal communication.

Hoeber S *et al.* (2016) Ultrasound-guided hip joint injections are more accurate than landmark-guided injections: a systematic review and meta-analysis. *Br J Sports Med.* **50** (7): 392–396.

Huang Z *et al.* (2015) Effectiveness of ultrasound guidance on intraarticular and peri-articular joint injections: systematic review and meta-analysis of randomized trials. *Am J Phys Med Rehabil.* **94** (10): 775–783.

Jones A *et al* (1993) Importance of placement of intra-articular steroid injections. *BMJ.* **307**: 1329–1330.

Kneebone R (2004) *Teaching and learning basic skills using multimedia and models.* PhD Thesis.

Lebrun CM (2016) Ultrasound-guided corticosteroid injections for adhesive capsulitis more effective than placebo. *Evid Based Med.* **21** (2): 71.

Liddell WG *et al* (2005) Joint and soft tissue injections: a survey of general practitioners. *Rheumatol.* **44**: 1043–1046.

Ryans I *et al* (2005) A randomised controlled trial of intra-articular triamcinolone and/ or physiotherapy in shoulder capsulitis. *Rheumatol.* **44**: 529–535.

Sage W *et al.* (2013) The clinical and functional outcomes of ultrasound-guided vs landmark-guided injections for adults with shoulder pathology: a systematic review and meta-analysis. *Rheumatology (Oxford).* **52** (4): 743–751.

Taylor J *et al.* (2016) Extracorporeal shockwave therapy (ESWT) for refractory Achilles tendinopathy: a prospective audit with 2-year follow up. *Foot (Edinb).* **26**: 23–29.

Thomas E *et al* (2005) Two pragmatic trials of treatment for shoulder disorders in primary care: generalisability, course and prognostic indicators. *Ann Rheum Dis.* **64**: 1056–1061.

Van der Heijden GJ *et al* (1996) Steroid injection for shoulder disorders: a systematic review of randomised clinical trails. *Br J Gen Pract.* **46**: 309–316.

Van der Heijden GJ *et al* (1997) Physiotherapy for patients with soft tissue shoulder disorders: A systematic review of randomised clinical trials. *BMJ.* **315**: 25–30.

Van der Windt DA *et al* (1995) The efficacy of NSAIDs for shoulder complaints. *J Clin Epidemiol.* **48**: 691–704.

Van der Windt DA *et al* (1997) *Steroid Injection or Physiotherapy for Capsulitis of the Shoulder: a Randomised Clinical Trial in Primary Care.* Privately published.

Winters JC *et al* (1997) Comparison of physiotherapy, manipulation and steroid injection for treating shoulder complaints in general practice: a randomised single blind study. *BMJ.* **314**: 1320–1325.

Wu T *et al.* (2015) Ultrasound-guided versus blind subacromial-subdeltoid bursa injection in adults with shoulder pain: a systematic review and meta-analysis. *Semin Arthritis Rheum.* **45** (3): 374–378.

CHAPTER 2

Joint and soft tissue corticosteroid injection: what is the evidence?

INTRODUCTION

The use of corticosteroid injections in the treatment of soft tissue and joint inflammatory conditions is now commonplace in both primary and secondary care.

Such procedures aid in the diagnosis and the treatment of a wide range of musculoskeletal pathologies and are a remarkable adjunct to both pharmacological and physical therapies with regards to a patient's rehabilitation and recovery.

Despite the overwhelming anecdotal practice-based experience that suggests that such treatments are effective, the evidence base is fairly limited.

This chapter aims to review the evidence for corticosteroid joint and soft tissue injection.

UPPER LIMB

Shoulder

Within the primary care setting shoulder complaints are common and account for one in every 170 adult consultations. With an average-sized GP practice, one may see up to 30 patients a year. Pathologies include instability in the younger adult, impingement (rotator cuff tendinopathy) in the 25–50-year-old age group and frozen shoulder in the older diabetic patient. Inflammatory shoulder joint problems are less common.

A careful history and examination will enable one to diagnose most of these clinically. Where there is diagnostic doubt, radiographs and blood tests will help aid in the diagnostic process. It cannot be stressed enough that the diagnostic process is extremely important, especially if a steroid injection is contemplated, as this will be more effective when injected into the appropriate anatomical compartment, for example, glenohumeral, acromioclavicular or subacromial space.

A Cochrane review published in 2003 specifically looked at the efficacy of corticosteroid injection for shoulder pain of various aetiologies. The review was based on the results of 26 trials. For rotator cuff disease, subacromial steroid injection was demonstrated to have a small benefit over placebo; however, no benefit of subacromial steroid injection over NSAID was demonstrated based upon the results of three trials. For adhesive capsulitis, two trials suggested an early benefit of intra-articular steroid injection over placebo, and one trial suggested a short-term benefit of intra-articular corticosteroid injection over physiotherapy in the short term. The authors concluded that subacromial corticosteroid injection for cuff disease and intra-articular injection for adhesive capsulitis may be beneficial, although their effect may be small and not well maintained. Important issues that remain to be clarified include whether the accuracy of needle placement, anatomical site, frequency, dose and type of corticosteroid influences efficacy.[1]

Previous reviews published in 1996[2] and 1998[3] analysed the findings of 16 and 31 trials, respectively (10 looked specifically at corticosteroid injection). The authors concluded that there was little evidence in favour of supporting the use of any intervention in the management of shoulder pain, and that further prospective randomised trials were required.

A study carried out specifically in the primary care setting, comparing cortico-steroid injection and physical therapy for shoulder pain, claimed a 77% success rate with surgery as opposed to 46% with physical therapy. A major limitation, however, was the lack of specific diagnoses.[4]

Elbow

Elbow pain is a common cause of presentation to the primary care physician. The most common pathologies seen relate to tendinopathy at the common flexor and extensor origins, namely medial and lateral epicondylitis, or golfer's or tennis elbow. The term epicondylitis is a bit of a misnomer as the pathophysiology is degenerative rather than inflammatory.[5] Despite this, corticosteroid has been shown to be a useful treatment when combined with other non-invasive measures. Hay et al[6] randomised patients with lateral epicondylitis to three treatment arms: placebo, oral NSAID and corticosteroid injections. They found that the best short-term (4-week) symp-tomatic improvements occurred in the corticosteroid injection group. At the 1-year follow-up, patient outcomes were similar among the three groups.

Medial epicondylitis or 'golfer's elbow' is less common than lateral epicondylitis but is often observed in labourers and those involved in repetitive wrist flexion and throwing athletes. Stahl et al[7] showed symptom improvement following corticosteroid administration at 6 weeks compared with controls, but no difference at 3 or 12 months.

Hand

The joints of the hand and wrist along with soft tissue structures are sites for injection for a variety of pathologies, including inflammatory arthropathy and osteoarthritis, tenosynovitis, carpal tunnel syndrome and triggering.

A clinical observational study involving 83 patients with trapeziometacarpal osteoarthritis showed 15% of patients had significant pain relief at 6 months, and nearly half had pain relief for more than 3 months, with a median response to injection of 2.5 months.[8]

Other studies have shown variable results. A randomised controlled trial (RCT) with 40 patients with first carpometacarpal osteoarthritis showed no benefit from intra-articular steroid injection compared with a placebo at 4, 12 and 24 weeks, based on joint stiffness, pain and visual analogue scale (VAS) scores.[9]

Median nerve entrapment within the carpal tunnel – carpal tunnel syndrome – is the commonest nerve entrapment syndrome, affecting up to 4% of the general population. A Cochrane review published in 2007 showed that local corticoste-roid injection provided greater symptom improvement at 1 month compared with placebo injection and provided significant clinical improvement over oral steroids for up to 3 months.[10]

A clinical review of the efficacy of steroid injection for the treatment of trig-ger finger summarised the results from two clinical trials involving a total of

63 patients. The authors concluded that better short-term results were achieved with a combination injection of corticosteroid and local anaesthetic compared with local anaesthetic alone. One of the studies showed that this effect was seen as far as 4 months post injection.[11]

Corticosteroid injection (and local anaesthetic) for de Quervain's tenosynovitis has been shown to be superior to splinting with thumb spica at 1 and 6 days following injection. The study group was small, however. The duration of follow-up was short and limited to pregnant and lactating women only.[12]

LOWER LIMB

Hip

Trochanteric bursitis, or greater trochanteric pain syndrome, is a common problem seen by primary care and sports physicians, characterised by lateral hip pain exacerbated by movement. Most cases respond to conservative measures, including lifestyle modification, physical therapy and weight loss, in conjunction with non-steroidal anti-inflammatories and corticosteroid injection.

A systematic review from 2011[13] reviewed nine studies that examined the effect of corticosteroid injection as the primary treatment modality. Studies measured outcomes using the VAS and showed a mean score improvement of 2.8. Subject improvement and a return to baseline activity were observed in between 49% and 100% of study patients. Most patients required a single injection. However, in some cases, several injections were required for on-going symptoms. Despite the results from this review and encouraging results from older studies, which lack validated outcome scoring, more robust randomised clinical trials are required to elucidate the benefit of corticosteroid administration over other treatment modalities.

Hip/knee

A study from the Mayo clinic, Rochester, MN, USA, reviewed 1188 patients in the primary care setting. Patients undergoing joint and bursal injections around the knee, hip and shoulder were evaluated using validated pre- and post-procedural pain scores and QOL (quality of life) – both physical and mental – assessment tools. They found, at 4 weeks, that there was a statistically significant improvement in pain and physical QOL scores at all injection sites. Interestingly, mental QOL scores improved specifically in women and in those greater than 60 years of age.[14] As with much of the published data, the limitation would be the lack of mid- and longer-term follow-up.

Foot

Plantar fasciitis is a common, and often debilitating, condition resulting in severe heel pain (often medial) that worsens with weight bearing or running. Conservative therapies are the mainstay of treatment. Corticosteroids are generally reserved for patients who fail a period of conservative treatment. A RCT with 65 patients randomised to placebo or corticosteroid injection showed a clear benefit of corticosteroid over placebo at both 6 and 12 weeks.[15] Another systematic review showed that compared with local anaesthetic alone a cortisone injection plus local anaesthetic may be more effective at improving pain scores in people with heel pain at 1 month. The use of corticosteroids was associated with a higher incidence of plantar fascia rupture, however.[16]

WHAT SHOULD WE INJECT?

The choice of corticosteroid injection is largely down to personal preference and while there is little good quality evidence to guide selection of a particular corticosteroid, knowledge of the pharmacokinetics of the various preparations can help guide selection for the appropriate clinical situation.

Insoluble steroid preparations have a more prolonged duration of action by allowing the preparation to remain at the injected site for longer; this does, however, theoretically increase the risk of local soft tissue complications.

As a general rule, low-solubility preparations are better suited to intra-articular injections, while a more soluble compound with a shorter duration of action is better reserved for soft tissue placement, with the theoretical benefit of fewer soft tissue side effects.

HOW OFTEN DO WE INJECT?

Data from studies in patients with rheumatoid arthritis suggest it is safe to perform multiple repeat injections on the same joint.[17] The recommended interval between repeat injections should be at least 3 months.[18] However, it is important to take into consideration one's clinical judgment, the underlying disease process, past response to injection, the availability of other treatment options and patient choice in deciding on injection frequency.

IS IT SAFE TO INJECT IN THE DIABETIC PATIENT?

A clinical concern is the use of steroids in patients with underlying diabetes mellitus. A single intra-articular injection has been shown to have little or no effect on systemic blood glucose control.[19] A periarticular or soft tissue injection, however, can cause elevations in blood glucose for up to 21 days. Therefore, close glucose control is advised in diabetics following such injections.[20,21]

WHAT IS THE ROLE OF IMAGE-GUIDED INJECTION?

The use of ultrasound as an adjunct is well established in the treatment of many joint and soft tissue pathologies; it enables the clinician to make a confident diagnosis and a more appropriate management plan. Imaging also has the added benefit of accurately locating areas of anatomical abnormality. Areas of anatomical abnormality, sites of maximal inflammation, fluid or hypervascularity can then be accurately targeted with an injection directly into or around the abnormal area or areas. Imaging can also visualise the surrounding structures and may help diagnose an underlying cause of the problem, for example, an underlying structural abnormality or a predisposing anatomical variant.

Imaging is not without its drawbacks, however. It has a significant cost implication and can result in a delay in the diagnosis and treatment of a condition that could, potentially, be dealt with swiftly and effectively in the primary care setting. Such delays in treatment can cause undue stress, potential time off work and reduction in QOL.

The accuracy of steroid placement has been shown to be associated with improved clinical outcomes in a number of studies.[22,23] The anatomical accuracy of blind injections was shown to be variable with successful placement seen between 37% and 52% of patients. Accurate subacromial injection placement was unsurprisingly less common as its position can be variable and was observed in only 29%.[22]

In 2009, a 148-patient RCT assessed the outcomes of ultrasound versus palpation-guided intra-articular needle placement. It showed that ultrasound methods resulted in a 58.5% reduction in absolute pain scores and a 75% reduction in significant pain compared with palpation methods at 2 weeks. Ultrasound also increased detection of effusion by 200% and volume of fluid aspirated by 37% compared with palpation.[24] The same group also published longer-term follow-up data (6 months) from 244 patients undergoing either ultrasound or palpation-guided intra-articular joint injection for inflammatory arthropathy. They showed not only a statistically significant reduction of pain scores at 2 weeks and 6 months, but an increase in the responder rate, a decrease in the non-responder rate and a 32% increase in therapeutic duration with ultrasound. Interestingly, in favour of the ultrasound group, cost-analysis calculations showed an 8% reduction ($7) in cost/patient/year and a 33% ($64) reduction in cost/responder/year for a hospital outpatient.[25]

Despite the number of studies favouring ultrasound-guided corticosteroid placement, a systematic review in 2012 compared the efficacy of image-guided (ultrasound) versus landmark-guided versus systemic intramuscular injection for the treatment of shoulder pain. The data of five trials were included in the review – four studies compared image-guided subacromial injection with blind injection, and one compared image-guided injection with systemic buttock injection. They found that, overall, no significant differences in pain were observed between groups at 1 or 2 weeks.[26]

While some studies show and favour the use of ultrasound-guided over 'blind' joint/soft tissue injection, there is no overwhelming clear-cut scientific proof.

Imaging has an important role to play in the management of bone and soft tissue disorders.

From a diagnostic point of view, it allows one to be more confident of the actual diagnosis and should be mandatory in cases of failed or refractory 'blind injection'.

Image-guided injection also allows accurate injection into areas of visible abnormality. Because of the inherent spatial resolution of ultrasound, small structures can be targeted easily (such as the subacromial bursae, which is in the order of a few millimetres when not distended). Such accuracy is obviously not permissible when relying on landmarks alone.

REFERENCES

1 Buchbinder R *et al* (2003) Corticosteroid injections for shoulder pain. *Cochrane Database Syst Rev.* **1**: CD004016.

2 van der Heijden GJ *et al* (1996) Steroid injection for shoulder disorders: a systematic review of randomised clinical trials. *Br J Gen Pract.* **46** (406): 309–316.

3 Green S *et al* (1998) Systematic review of randomised controlled trials of interventions for painful shoulder: selection criteria, outcome assessment, and efficacy. *BMJ.* **316** (7128): 354–360.

4 van der Windt *et al* (1998) Effectiveness of corticosteroid injection versus physiotherapy for the treatment of a painful stiff shoulder in primary care: randomised trial. *Br Med J.* **317**: 1292–1296.

5 Kraushaar BS and Nirschl RP (1999) Tendinosis of the elbow (tennis elbow): clinical features and findings of histological, immunohistochemical, and electron microscopy studies. *J Bone Joint Surg Am.* **81** (2): 259–278.

6 Hay EM *et al* (1999) Pragmatic randomised controlled trial of local corticosteroid injection and naproxen for treatment of lateral epicondylitis of elbow in primary care. *BMJ.* **319** (7215): 964–968.

7 Stahl S and Kaufman T (1997) The efficacy of an injection of steroids for medial epicondylitis: a prospective study of sixty elbows. *J Bone Joint Surg Am.* **79** (11): 1648–1652.

8 Swindells MG *et al* (2010) The benefit of radiologically-guided steroid injections for trapeziometacarpal osteoarthritis. *Ann R Coll Surg Engl.* **92** (8): 680–684.

9 Meenagh GK *et al* (2004) A randomised controlled trial of intra-articular corticosteroid injection of the carpometacarpal joint of the thumb in osteoarthritis. *Ann Rheum Dis.* **63** (10): 1260–1263.

10 Marshall S *et al* (2007) Local corticosteroid injection for carpal tunnel syndrome. *Cochrane Database Syst Rev* **2**: CD001554.

11 Peters-Veluthamaningal C *et al* (2009) Corticosteroid injection for trigger finger in adults. *Cochrane Database Syst Rev.* **1**: CD005617.

12 Peters-Veluthamaningal C *et al* (2009) Corticosteroid injection for de Quervain's tenosynovitis. *Cochrane Database Syst Rev.* **3**: CD005616.

13 Lustenberger D *et al* (2011) Efficacy of treatment of trochanteric bursitis: a systematic review. *Clin J Sport Med.* **21**(5): 447–453.

14 Bhagra A *et al* (2013) Efficacy of musculoskeletal injections by primary care providers in the office: a retrospective cohort study. *Int J Gen Med.* **6**: 237–243.

15 Ball EM *et al* (2013) Steroid injection for inferior heel pain: a randomized controlled trial. *Ann Rheum Dis.* **72**: 996–1002.

16 Landorf KB and Menz HB (2008) Plantar heel pain and fasciitis. *Clin Evid (Online).* **pii**: 1111.

17 Combe B (2007) Early rheumatoid arthritis: strategies for prevention and management. *Best Pract Res Clin Rheumatol.* **21** (1): 27–42.

18   Raynauld JP *et al* (2003) Safety and efficacy of long-term intraarticular steroid injections in osteoarthritis of the knee: a randomized, double-blind, placebo-controlled trial. *Arthritis Rheum.* **48** (2): 370–377.

19 Habib GS and Abu-Ahmad R (2006) Lack of effect of corticosteroid injection at the shoulder joint on blood glucose levels in diabetic patients. *Clin Rheumatol.* **26** (4): 566–558.

20 Younes M *et al* (2007) Systemic effects of epidural and intra-articular glucocorticoid injections in diabetic and non-diabetic patients. *Joint Bone Spine* 74 (5): 472–476.

21 Wang AA and Hutchinson DT (2006) The effect of corticosteroid injection for trigger finger on blood glucose level in diabetic patients. *J Hand Surg Am.* **31** (6): 979–981.

22 Jones A *et al* (1993) Importance of placement of intra-articular steroid injections. *BMJ.* **307** (6915): 1329–1330.

23 Eustace JA *et al* (1997) Comparison of the accuracy of steroid placement with clinical outcome in patients with shoulder symptoms. *Ann Rheum Dis.* **56** (1): 59–63.

24 Sibbitt WL *et al* (2009) Does sonographic needle guidance affect the clinical outcome of intraarticular injections? *J Rheumatol.* **36** (9): 1892–1902.

25 Sibbitt WL Jr *et al* (2011) A randomized controlled trial of the cost-effectiveness of ultrasound-guided intraarticular injection of inflammatory arthritis. *J Rheumatol.* **38** (2): 252–263.

26 Bloom JE *et al* (2012) Image-guided versus blind glucocorticoid injection for shoulder pain. Cochrane Database Syst Rev. Issue 8. Art. No.: CD009147.

CHAPTER 3

Medico-legal issues, complications and consent

INTRODUCTION

Because steroids have, over the years, been notable because of the number of undesirable side effects, as well as their magical clinical effects, their prescription and use have come under severe scrutiny by the public at large. To this end, the legal professions on both sides of the Atlantic have enjoyed a bonanza of medical litigation, much of which has been spurious. Nevertheless, media attention has been prolific, and words of caution to the medical profession will not be untoward in this manual.

Steroids are potent anti-inflammatory drugs but, at the same time, inappropriate or overuse may well spell disaster for a patient. There are several concepts that should be considered, which should be incorporated into the practicing physician's normal daily routine.

TECHNIQUE OF THE PROCEDURE

Demonstrating careful and efficient management in the treatment room creates a good impression. Washing the hands, wearing sterile gloves, using single-dose vials and having clean surroundings are all important. Sterilising the operation site and putting an Elastoplast® plaster over the injection site after the procedure are both evidence of care and go a long way to ensuring that the patient is receiving the best possible attention.

The images in this book are included to illustrate the techniques and it is advised that practitioners consider the use of sterile gloves when performing injections.

UNTOWARD COMPLICATIONS OF STEROID INJECTION

Lipodystrophy

When steroid is inadvertently injected subcutaneously, lipodystrophy may occur. This will result in dimpling of the skin, which may well upset a patient, especially if they have not been warned beforehand. Because these lesions are quite superficial, this effect occurs more commonly after injections for tennis and golfer's elbow. Although the more potent steroids have the reputation of being susceptible in this respect, it is wise to warn patients of this possibility. In the author's opinion, any subcutaneous injection of steroid may cause lipodystrophy.

Injections undertaken with image guidance are very likely to make this complication less significant, as inadvertent subcutaneous injection can be avoided in most cases.

Loss of skin pigment

Injecting steroid subcutaneously in patients with dark skin may occasionally leave a small area of pigment loss. Again, it is wise to warn of this possibility and pre-empt any cause for subsequent complaint.

Repeat injections at the same site are not recommended. For example, there have been cases of tendon rupture of the patellar tendon following repeated injection of the infrapatellar bursa of the knee joint. Practitioners should be aware of this complication.

Other tendons known to rupture are the Achilles, of which mention has already been made, the bicipital (long head of the biceps), which is known to rupture spontaneously, and the palmar flexor tendons. In all of these cases, caution is advised in the use of steroid injection.

A 2005 review (58 references) of injectable steroids in modern practice suggested that corticosteroids of low solubility are thought to have the longest duration of action. Intra-articular steroids have been shown to be safe and effective for repeated use (every 3 months) for up to 2 years, with no detectable joint space narrowing seen. The accuracy of injections affects their outcomes. Post-injection flare, facial flushing and skin and fat atrophy are the most common side effects. Systemic complications of injectable steroids are rare.[1]

Hyperglycaemia

Intra-articular and soft tissue steroid injections have been shown to elevate blood sugar in diabetic patients, commencing after a few hours and lasting for several days. However, although these small increases in glycaemia are statistically significant, they are, generally, not considered clinically significant.[2,3]

Infection

The incidence of septic arthritis is rare, but it is a recognised complication, despite aseptic technique and image guidance. The patient should be consented for such complications (albeit rare) as the significances of these complications are very significant.

Rates between 1:3000 and 1:50,000 are quoted in the literature.

PAIN AFTER INJECTION

These injection procedures are often painful at the time of injection. Many will give rise to pain after the local anaesthetic effect has worn off, sometimes for up to 48 hours after the injection. It is, therefore, wise to warn every patient of this possibility, as forewarned is forearmed. Simple advice should be given to take appropriate analgesic tablets: 2 × 500 mg paracetamol tablets 4-hourly as required while the pain lasts.

Pain may well be more significant after blind injections where steroid is inadvertently injected into muscle. With this regard, it may be appropriate to consider image-guided injection to reduce this unwanted complication, which may reduce the benefit of such an intervention.

More importantly, the development of pain increasing in severity some 48 hours after injection may herald the very serious complication of a septic arthritis. Warning the patient of this very rare complication is mandatory as part of consent, and informing the patient to return immediately to the doctor or seek medical advice for reassessment in such an event may well avoid a serious cause for litigation.

Potential complications from injection

- Hypersensitivity – local or systemic.
- Tissue atrophy, nodule formation and skin hypopigmentation.
- Tendon rupture.
- Infection – local or systemic.
- Post-injection flare of symptoms.
- Osteonecrosis/steroid arthropathy.
- Facial flushing – usually 24–72 hours post injection and predominantly women.
- Menstrual irregularity.
- Elevated blood sugar in diabetic patients.
- Fainting.

INFORMED CONSENT

Advice, provided with consent, is an essential part of the recognition of patient autonomy and the right to choose. Healthcare practitioners should recognise the need to involve patients in decisions about their care. Whenever possible, you must be satisfied, before you provide treatment, that the patient has understood what is proposed and why, is appropriately informed about the balance of risk and benefit and has given consent.

It is important to ensure that:

1 The patient has the right information to make a decision.
2 The information has been presented in a way the patient can understand.
3 The patient has shared in the process of decision-making and agrees with the outcome.

'Prudent doctor/prudent patient'

The courts used to apply the 'prudent doctor' principle. This is where the doctor weighs the risk of a certain complication against the risk of putting a patient off the necessary treatment. Complications with a very low incidence were generally considered not worth mentioning, unless they would have serious ramifications. The shift in recent years has been to the 'prudent patient' model, which reflects what the average patient would want to know about potential risks.

Implied consent

It is important to explain to patients the potential risks and benefits of a particular procedure. In the majority of injections, the risk involved would be very low. In these cases, the prior consent of the patient will be obtained at the time of the procedure. The patient's actions at the time of this procedure will indicate whether the patient is content for this to proceed.

Express consent

Judgement is required as to when express consent must be obtained and the degree of detail appropriate to a discussion with the patient about a particular procedure. Different procedures may involve different explanatory processes by different practitioners; however, variation should not to detract from the fact that consent is required before the procedure is initiated. Express consent can be given either verbally or in writing.

Injection procedures

Injection procedures require particular attention in obtaining the express consent of the patient. In a planned procedure, the patient should receive information, verbally or in writing, in sufficient time before the procedure to consider it and to consult others if they so wish. Ideally, the patient should have provided consent confirmed at a separate discussion prior to the procedure.

Written consent

The General Medical Council suggests that written consent should be taken in cases where:

1 The injection is complex and involves significant risk or side effects.
2 Complications may result in significant consequences for the patient's employment, social or personal life.

Consent must be given freely without pressure from anyone. If consent is given under duress, consent will be deemed invalid.

If the patient asks for your opinion as a doctor involved in their care, then it should be given on history, accurately and clearly given. This advice should be based on what is in the best interest of the patient, without knowledge of the risks and benefits involved.

The Mental Capacity Act 2005 (England and Wales) provides a framework to protect people who lack the mental capacity to make some decisions for themselves. The Act makes it clear that you can take decisions in certain situations, and how you should go about this. It also allows people to plan ahead for a time when they may lack such mental capacity.

Documentation of consent

Patients have a right to information about the condition and the treatment options available.

The amount of information you provide each patient will vary according to factors such as the nature of the condition and the complexity of the procedure.

Information should be given, including:

1 The diagnosis and prognosis.
2 Any uncertainty about the diagnosis or prognosis.

3 Options for treating or managing the condition.

4 The purpose of any proposed treatment.

5 The potential benefits, risks and the likelihood of success.

It is important to emphasise that patients cannot give valid consent unless they understand what they have been told. The presentation of information to patients must, therefore, take into account the patient's values, culture, language, background, age and mental ability.

Patient literature should give clear information. Ideally, information should be given to the patient before the time of their procedure, and it is advisable to prepare patient information leaflets to address this important aspect of consent.

It is very important that records are created and kept following an injection procedure.

REFERENCES

1 Cole B et al (2005) Injectable corticosteroids in modern practice. *J Am Acad Orthop Surg.* **13** (1): 37–46.

2 Papadopoulos PJ and Edison JD (2009) The clinical picture: soft tissue atrophy after corticosteroid injection. *Cleve Clin J Med.* **76** (6): 373–374.

3 Kallock E et al (2010) Clinical inquiries. Do intra-articular steroid injections affect glycemic control in patients with diabetes? *J Fam Pract.* **59** (12): 709–710.

FURTHER READING

Alexander JW et al (2011) Updated recommendations for control of surgical site infections. *Ann Sur.* **253** (6): 1082–1093.

Brinks A et al (2010) Adverse effects of extra-articular corticosteroid injections: a systematic review. *Musculoskeletal Dis.* **11**: 206.

Cawley PJ and Morris IM (1992) A study to compare the efficacy of two methods of skin preparation prior to joint injection. *Brit J Rheumatol.* **31** (12): 847–848.

General Medical Council. Consent: Patients and doctors making decisions together. http://www.gmc-uk.org/guidance/ethical_guidance/consent_guidance_index.asp [accessed on 8/10/18].

Hemani ML and Herbert LH (2009) Skin preparation for the prevention of surgical site infection: which agent is best? *Rev Urol.* **11** (4): 190–195.

McGarry J and Daruwalla Z (2011) The efficacy, accuracy and complications of corticosteroid injections of the knee joint. *Knee Surg Sports TraumatolArthrosc.* **19** (10): 1649.

Mental Capacity Act 2005. http://www.legislation.gov.uk/ukpga/2005/9/contents [accessed on 8/10/18].

Unglaub F et al (2005) Necrotizing fasciitis following therapeutic injection in a shoulder joint [in German]. *Orthopade.* **34** (3): 250–252.

CHAPTER 4

The challenge of recognising and managing inflammatory arthritis

INTRODUCTION

The indication for an injection is often an inflamed joint. This can be the first sign of a more diffuse inflammatory arthritis. Although this book is primarily aimed at enabling the reader to inject joints with confidence and good technique, it is also important for the injector to have some knowledge of this type of condition. The aim of this chapter is to give GPs, nurse specialists and healthcare professionals guidance on the diagnosis and management of inflammatory arthritis.

BACKGROUND: THE BURDEN OF INFLAMMATORY DISEASE

Inflammatory arthritis encompasses several different pathologies, the most common of which is rheumatoid arthritis (RA), and this will therefore be the main focus of this chapter. Other forms of persistent inflammatory arthritis include the seronegative spondyloarthropathies, namely ankylosing spondylitis, psoriatic arthritis, enteropathic arthritis and reactive arthritis. Acute inflammatory arthritis also includes gout and pseudogout, which typically present with discrete attacks.

RA is a chronic, autoimmune, inflammatory disorder, which primarily targets the synovium. It causes severe pain, swelling and inflammation of joints. RA typically affects the small joints of the hands and feet, usually in a symmetrical distribution. However, any synovial joint can be affected. It can lead to considerable joint destruction and disability. Women are approximately three times more likely to be affected than men. The peak age of onset is 40–50 years.[1] The prevalence of RA is estimated at 580,000 people in England, with an incidence of 26,000 new cases diagnosed each year. The economic disease burden is huge, costing the National Health Service (NHS) £580 million/year. There is an even greater cost to the UK economy, with an estimated £1.8 billion in sick leave and work-related disability.[2]

Prompt recognition and referral to a specialist can help lessen the individual and economic burden. The landmark Cobra trial demonstrates that early diagnosis (within 3 months from symptom onset) and initiation of treatment is important for achieving long-term disease remission. Treating within this window of opportunity has led to favourable outcomes with higher rates of maintaining remission and preventing joint erosion.[3] Unfortunately, due to significant diagnostic challenges and referral pathways, the average time from symptom onset to initiation of treatment is typically nine months.[2]

CHALLENGES TO DIAGNOSIS

There are several barriers to the timely diagnosis and treatment of inflammatory arthritis. There is often significant delay from symptom onset to presentation to the GP. This can be due to a number of factors, including the patient's perceived cause of the symptoms and the presentation, location and experience of these symptoms, as well as GP-related drivers and barriers.[4]

Recognising the early stages of inflammatory arthritis can be challenging because signs of synovitis at this stage are often subtle. On average, a patient visits their

GP four times before referral to a specialist.[2] A gradual or stuttering onset of joint inflammation (palindromic arthritis), due to the intermittent nature of the symptoms, is often diagnosed later.

Another critical barrier can be the arrangement of a timely appointment with a specialist. The introduction of early arthritis clinics in many rheumatology departments has proven very effective at reducing this cause of delay.[5] These clinics have been organised specifically for patients who have developed recent onset arthritis. They are often alongside nurse specialist clinics so that patients are diagnosed, counselled and started on disease-modifying antirheumatic drug (DMARD) medications promptly in a single visit.

HOW TO DIAGNOSE

Clinical findings

RA is a clinical diagnosis. A typical history will involve pain, stiffness and swelling of the joints in a pattern described earlier. The degree and timing of stiffness is important; patients often describe significant early morning (>30 minutes) inactivity stiffness. A careful clinical examination is vital to search for signs of synovitis, which is felt as a tender, warm, boggy swelling of synovial joints. They may also have extra-articular features such as skin nodules, eye involvement (e.g. episcleritis), lung involvement (e.g. pulmonary fibrosis) and cardiac involvement (e.g. pericarditis).

Special investigations

Raised inflammatory markers and a positive rheumatoid factor (RF) can be helpful in supporting a clinical suspicion of inflammatory arthritis. However, do not be falsely reassured if they are normal. A mildly-raised RF is also commonly seen in smokers. As part of the diagnostic work up, it is important to test the patient for anti-citrullinated c-peptide (anti-CCP) in addition to RF. If either of these antibodies are positive, this indicates a more aggressive phenotype of RA.

In these cases, joint destruction and extra-articular manifestations are more likely. Checking baseline hand and feet radiographs are helpful in suspected cases of inflammatory arthritis. Not only do they give a valuable baseline for future comparison, but if erosions are present at this early stage, treatment can be prompt and aggressive.

MANAGEMENT

When persistent inflammatory arthritis is diagnosed, patients are treated with steroids (systemic, intramuscular or intra-articular) in the short term. This usually comprises a period of 4 to 8 weeks of systemic steroids in a tapering fashion. This gives rapid treatment of inflammation and rapid symptomatic relief.

For maintenance of disease remission, DMARDs such as methotrexate, leflunomide, sulfasalazine and hydroxychloroquine are used. These often require up to 12 weeks to take effect.

Methotrexate is the most commonly used DMARD and, providing there are no contraindications for its use, it is our first drug of choice for RA. All patients require blood testing (particularly to check renal, liver and bone marrow function) together with a chest radiograph prior to its use. Pulmonary function tests are also useful in patients with concurrent lung disease. A patient with a low total diffusion capacity (DLCO) will not have the lung reserve to compensate in the rare case of methotrexate pneumonitis. This drug should be avoided in such cases. Most centres employ a DMARD counselling service delivered by specialist nurses.

The evidence has shown that combination DMARD therapy is superior to monotherapy in inducing remission, maintaining remission and preventing erosion.[6] Therefore, two or more DMARDs are often combined from the outset. Early arthritis clinics are designed to have well-defined follow-up, often in a nurse-led clinic 6 weeks after commencing treatment. The purpose of this is to assess treatment response and tolerability of medications. Later, disease activity should be reassessed by a specialist clinician in order to measure the efficacy of the DMARDs used and determine future therapy. The disease activity score (DAS) is a composite score based on the number of tender joints, the number of swollen joints, a VAS score from the patient and the C-reactive protein/erythrocyte sedimentation rate. The DAS28 score (based on counting 28 joints) forms the basis of criteria for eligibility for biologic medications. In accordance with National Institute for Health and Care Excellence (NICE) criteria, if patients with RA have evidence of high disease activity (DAS28 >5.1) despite the use of two or more DMARDs (one of which being methotrexate, unless contraindicated), a patient may then progress to biological treatment.

These drugs have revolutionised the treatment of RA, achieving high rates of disease remission that were not possible prior to their inception. There is evidence that supports tight treatment control regimens with regular follow-ups in the treat-to-target initiative adopted in many rheumatology centres.[7]

Biological medications are immunosuppressive and therefore should be stopped temporarily should a patient develop symptoms or signs of infection. They can be restarted once the infection has been fully treated. It is important to remember that patients on immunosuppressive therapies can have atypical presentations of underlying infections.

INJECTING IN INFLAMMATORY ARTHRITIS

Treating disease flares often involves giving a short regimen of corticosteroid. This can be in the form of systemic, intramuscular or intra-articular steroid. Where a patient has few affected joints, the clinician can use the intra-articular route to avoid systemic side effects. It is important to always consider the possibility of septic arthritis, which is inherently more common in a damaged joint. Any suspicion of this will require consideration of aspiration and immediate referral to secondary care services.

CONCLUSION

Despite the significant challenges of diagnosing inflammatory arthritis, there have been considerable advances in our knowledge of the condition and the treatments used. Modern rheumatological practice involves aggressive early intervention with combination DMARD therapy. Biological medications have a pivotal role in severe active RA not responding to DMARDs. Hopefully, with greater awareness of the condition comes earlier diagnosis and treatment. With such huge benefits to be gained from early treatment, we cannot afford to miss this opportunity.

REFERENCES

1 West SG (2014) *Rheumatology Secrets*, 3rd edn. Mosby, St. Louis, USA. ISBN 0323037003.

2 Parliament publication http://www.publications.parliament.uk/pa/cm200910/cmselect/cmpubacc/46/46.pdf [accessed on 27/4/17].

3 Boers M *et al* (1997) Randomised comparison of combined step-down prednisolone, methotrexate and sulphasalazine with sulphasalazine alone in early rheumatoid arthritis. *Lancet.* **350**: 309–318.

4 Stack RJ *et al* (2012) Delays in help seeking at the onset of the symptoms of rheumatoid arthritis: a systematic synthesis of qualitative literature. *Ann Rheum Dis.* **71** (4): 493–497.

5 Monti S *et al* (2015) Rheumatoid arthritis treatment: the earlier the better to prevent joint damage. *RMD Open.* **1** (Suppl 1): e000057.

6 Goekoop-Ruiterman YP *et al* (2005) Clinical and radiographic outcomes of four different treatment strategies in patients with early rheumatoid arthritis (the BeSt study): a randomized, controlled trial. *Arthritis Rheum.* **52** (11): 3381–3390.

7 Grigor C *et al* (2004) Effect of a treatment strategy of tight control for rheumatoid arthritis (the TICORA study): A single-blind randomised controlled trial. *Lancet.* **364** (9430): 263–269.

CHAPTER 5

The shoulder

INTRODUCTION

There are many causes of pain in or around the shoulder joint. It is important to be accurate in diagnosis in order to determine those that will respond well to treatment with steroid injection.

It is an important concept to understand that many of the causes of pain related to the rotator cuff are degenerative in aetiology and the terminology describes the underlying pathology:

- *Tendinosis* is a misnomer, as inflammatory cells are rarely seen histologically.
- *Tendinopathy* is a clinical description referring to both acute and chronic conditions.
- *Tendinosis* refers to a non-inflammatory state with histological evidence of collagen disorganisation and necrosis.

The aetiology of tendinosis is multifactorial and commonly related to repeated episodes of microtrauma, with breakdown of collagen cross-linking. If repair is incomplete, it may progress to further injury and tendon failure.

Diagnoses to consider are as follows:

- Supraspinatus tendinosis (subscapularis, infraspinatus).
- Rotator cuff tear.
- Frozen shoulder (adhesive capsulitis).
- Subacromial bursitis.
- Bicipital tendinosis (long head of the biceps).
- Osteoarthritis of the acromioclavicular, or glenohumeral, joint.
- Acute arthropathies, for example, rheumatoid, psoriasis and other seronegative arthropathies.
- Calcific tendinosis.

PRESENTATION AND DIAGNOSIS

Shoulder pain occurs most commonly in the middle-aged or older-aged group of patients, and the incidence appears to plateau at about 45 years of age. Women are affected more frequently than men.

With improved and ready access to imaging, the clinician should not underestimate the value of radiographs. In patients over 60 with shoulder pain, osteoarthritis of the glenohumeral joint should not be overlooked, as this will not be diagnosed with an ultrasound scan. Patients who present with acute and often severe pain unrelated to movement should have a diagnosis of calcific tendinosis considered. A radiograph is diagnostic in this condition, which allows for options, including percutaneous barbotage under imaging, to effectively manage this condition, obviating the need for surgery in the majority.

It is important to note that acute onset of pain, especially if there is a history of trauma in patients under 45 years, should alert the clinician to a diagnosis of a rotator cuff tear, which usually primarily involves the supraspinatus, but may involve the subscapularis and biceps, if there is significant injury. Chondral injury should also be considered in the younger age groups, with or without a history of dislocation.

In this group of younger patients, referral to a shoulder surgeon should be considered, as outcomes are best with timely operative management.

In the past, the terminology has been loosely applied to these conditions but accurate diagnosis with ultrasound or MRI has changed this perspective.

A good example is that of 'subacromial bursitis' – the diagnosis often used in those patients presenting with a painful arc. It should be remembered that except in the context of inflammatory arthropathy, most pathology starts in the tendon, and if there is fluid in the bursa, then a tear of the underlying tendon should be actively considered. In the example of the shoulder, the supraspinatus acts as a watertight seal between the glenohumeral joint and the subacromial bursa. If there is fluid in the bursa, then it is likely this seal has been broken (i.e. there is a tear of the supraspinatus).

Frozen shoulder is a debilitating condition with an unclear aetiology; however, it can be a multifactorial condition. Presentation may be idiopathic, where no cause is identified, or be associated with a number of predisposing conditions:

1 Diabetes (10%–20% association). There is a 2–4 times increased risk for diabetics of developing frozen shoulder. Insulin-dependent diabetics have a 36% chance of developing it, 10% bilaterally, and the condition is more severe in diabetics.

2 Cardiac/lipid problems.

3 Epilepsy.

4 Endocrine abnormalities, particularly hypothyroidism.

5 Trauma.

6 Drugs.

7 Strong association with Dupuytren's contracture.

The following clinical phases are recognised:

- *Freezing phase*. Pain increases with movement and is often worse at night. There is a progressive loss of motion with increasing pain. This stage lasts approximately 2–9 months.

- *Frozen phase*. Pain begins to diminish; however, the range of motion is now much more limited, as much as 50% less than in the other arm. This stage may last 4–12 months.

- *Thawing phase*. The condition may begin to resolve. Most patients experience a gradual restoration of motion over the next 12–42 months.

Impingement syndrome is a diagnosis that has become fashionable in the past few years. It is characterised by pain at the lateral tip of the shoulder, on abduction of the arm, and is usually due to supraspinatus tendinosis. It is due to degeneration of the supraspinatus tendon, leading to reduced function and upward subluxation the humeral head due to deltoid acting unopposed. This, in turn, leads to narrowing of the subacromial space and 'snagging', or so-called impingement, on abduction.

PITFALLS IN DIAGNOSIS

Referred pain to the tip of the shoulder

Patients may complain of pain in the shoulder, which may be referred to the C5 dermatome by other conditions. These produce pain that are not necessarily related to muscle or tendon movement, for example:

- Bronchogenic carcinoma of the apex of the lung (Pancoast tumour).
- Cervical spine disc lesions or nerve entrapments.
- Heart problems.
- Diaphragmatic problems.
- Oesophageal conditions.

A high index of clinical suspicion is necessary to recognise a Pancoast tumour. This bronchogenic carcinoma affecting the apex of the lung may well produce pain referred to the tip of the shoulder. It is a great advantage in conditions such as these if the primary contact physician makes an early diagnosis. Where this does not happen, the patient with shoulder pain who is referred to a hospital rheumatological clinic may well wait up to 3 or 4 months for an outpatient appointment, by which time a late diagnosis of bronchogenic carcinoma can be catastrophic for the patient. In such instances, there is a strong case for general practitioners (GPs) who see their patients often at the onset of symptoms to be expert at diagnosing and treating these soft tissue disorders.

Polymyalgia rheumatica is another condition that presents early in the general practice setting. Doctors are only too well aware of the classical history of severe pain and stiffness affecting the hips and proximal thighs, together with the shoulders and upper arms, early in the morning. Occasionally, the onset may affect one shoulder only at the start of the disease, leading to some difficulty in differential diagnosis. What is a better achievement for the practitioner who diagnoses this condition at such an early stage? Being well aware of the presentation of all these disorders enhances the doctor's skill in diagnosis and early effective therapy. In this example, a simple erythrocyte sedimentation rate blood test may be all that is necessary to confirm the diagnosis of polymyalgia.

In diabetes, frozen shoulder occurs more frequently, and occasionally finding a patient whose condition has been slow to respond to steroid injection should alert one to this diagnosis, especially in a female aged over 50 years.

A good rule is to test the urine for sugar in a patient, more usually female, whose frozen shoulder problem has failed to improve with two or three steroid injections.

Pain referred to the deltoid insertion

Pain referred to the deltoid insertion halfway down the lateral side of the upper arm may occur in any of the rotator cuff pathologies and should not tempt the doctor to inject steroid at this site. The techniques for injection of the shoulder lesions described later in the text are always the ones that should be used.

FUNCTIONAL ANATOMY

Understanding the functional or clinical anatomy of the shoulder will ensure that a specific diagnosis is made, as well as give confidence in the skill of accurate injection. Lack of this knowledge has, in the past, prevented the practitioner from developing the confidence to know that the injecting needle is accurately sited. The aim in injecting the shoulder joint for rotator cuff lesions is to ensure that the needle enters the subacromial space. It is not necessary to attempt to place the needle point in the glenohumeral joint space and, in fact, this is extremely difficult using a non-guided technique.

The glenohumeral joint consists of the head of the humerus articulating with the glenoid fossa of the scapula. This shallow joint space is no more than 1.5 inches (3.8 cm) in length. The joint is held together by a rather loosely-applied voluminous capsule of fibrous tissue, which is considerably strengthened by the three tendons of the rotator cuff that blend with it anteriorly, posteriorly and superiorly, respectively, from the subscapularis, the infraspinatus together with teres minor, and the supraspinatus. The long head of the biceps tendon arises on the superior glenoid tubercle within the capsule of the joint and becomes covered by its own synovial sheath as it lies superiorly in the capsule. It leaves the joint space through an opening in the capsule, passing over the bicipital groove, which lies on the anterolateral surface of the head of the humerus, to join the short head of the biceps muscle anteriorly over the upper arm.

The subscapularis lies anteriorly, and internally (medially) rotates the arm; the infraspinatus (lies posteriorly) and teres minor together externally (laterally) rotate and the supraspinatus (lies superiorly) abducts the arm to 90 degrees ('the painful arc').

Because these tendons blend with the capsule of the shoulder joint, it is only necessary to inject into the space enclosed by the joint capsule – anatomically, this is the subacromial space – in order to bathe the soft tissue lesions in steroid and lidocaine, which effect resolution of the pain.

The role steroids have in effective management of a predominately degenerative condition remains largely an unsolved mystery.

Contrary to popular belief, it is not necessary to inject into the glenohumeral joint space itself.

The acromioclavicular joint

This is a small plane joint or synostosis where the lateral end of the clavicle articulates with the acromion process of the scapula. The capsular ligament is strengthened by the acromioclavicular ligament. There is a very small joint space that will admit 0.2–0.5 ml of injection fluid. Acromioclavicular pain is often overlooked as the cause of pain and a meticulous clinical examination will avoid this pitfall.

Note that bicipital tendinosis, which is a tenosynovitis of the sheath of this tendon, and osteoarthritis of the acromioclavicular joint, both common causes of shoulder pain, must be injected as described later for each particular condition. Failure to accurately diagnose and treat these disorders specifically contributes to the lack of success in shoulder injection to which some commentators refer.

EXAMINATION OF THE SHOULDER

An understanding of the functional anatomy of the shoulder allows a simple routine examination of the shoulder joint, which will accurately determine the source of the pain.

First, assess the cervical spine for the normal range of movements and to ascertain that no pain is referred from the neck to the shoulder. With the patient standing up, check:

- Forward flexion – ask the patient to bend the head forward as far as possible.
- Backward flexion – bend the head backwards as far as possible.
- Head rotation – rotate the head fully to right and then left, and (subjectively) measure any deficit in degrees.
- Lateral flexion – side bending to right and left sides.

Note any restrictions to these movements and whether any of these movements cause pain in the affected shoulder.

With the patient stripped to the waist, inspect both shoulders to exclude any joint swellings, effusion, signs of arthritis or subacromial impingement. Test for local points of tenderness. Tenderness of the shoulder over the bicipital tendon lying in the bicipital groove may suggest bicipital tendinosis, whereas tenderness palpated over the lateral tip of the shoulder may alert the examiner to the possibility of supraspinatus pathology.

Next, examine the full range of active movements. With the patient standing, ask him to do the following:

- Abduct both arms to 90 degrees with the palms facing the ceiling. This movement is performed by the supraspinatus. (The 'painful arc' is a term first described by James Cyriax as meaning pain in shoulder on active abduction of the arm). Restriction = supraspinatus tendinosis.
- Next, place both hands on the back of the head (the occiput). This is external rotation and is performed by the infraspinatus. Restriction = infraspinatus tendinosis.
- Now bring both arms behind the chest and raise the thumbs as high as possible. This movement is internal rotation and is performed by the subscapularis. Restriction = subscapularis tendinosis.

Note any pain or restriction of any of these rotator cuff movements. If all these movements are painful or restricted, the diagnosis of frozen shoulder is implied.

Note the pain caused by any of the specific movements that are reproduced on testing the resisted movements, which will indicate the tendon involved.

Passive movement of the shoulder with one hand placed over the joint may reveal any crepitus present in pericapsulitis (frozen shoulder). This condition is characteristically associated with loss of abduction relating to the underlying pathology affecting the rotator interval.

Diagnosis of any lesion is then confirmed by checking the resisted movements. A diagnosis of tendinosis (repetitive strain) may only be confirmed when pain and restricted movement are demonstrated on testing the resisted movements of the tendon.

In the diagnosis of soft tissue lesions, always remember to examine the:

1 ACTIVE movements.
2 RESISTED movements.
3 PASSIVE movements.

WHAT THE PAIN MEANS (SEE FIGURE 5.1)

Pain on resisted abduction

The patient abducts both arms up to 90 degrees while the examiner applies counterpressure to this movement. If this causes pain, the diagnosis is supraspinatus tendinosis or, possibly, a tear. In this condition, radiographic examination of the shoulder may reveal calcification in the substance of the supraspinatus tendon. This is no contraindication to steroid injection, which is very effective.

If pain is experienced when the arms are raised in the range from 90 degrees (horizontal) to 180 degrees (vertical), this suggests osteoarthritis of the acromio-clavicular joint (*see* p. 34).

Resisted external rotation

With both elbows pressed into the ribs and with the arms flexed at 90 degrees pointing forwards, the patient pushes the forearms and hands outwards against resistance. Pain indicates infraspinatus tendinosis, although isolated tears or pathology affecting infraspinatus are rare and usually follow significant tears affecting supraspinatus.

Resisted internal rotation

With both elbows tucked into the ribs and both arms flexed at 90 degrees, the patient presses the hands inwards against resistance. Pain indicates subscapularis tendinosis.

Resisted supination and flexion of the forearm

The patient flexes the forearms against resistance or supinates the wrist against resistance with the elbow bent to 90 degrees. Pain felt at the tip of the shoulder implies bicipital tendinosis. An alternative test is to resist forward movement of the arm with the elbow extended, producing pain at the tip of the shoulder.

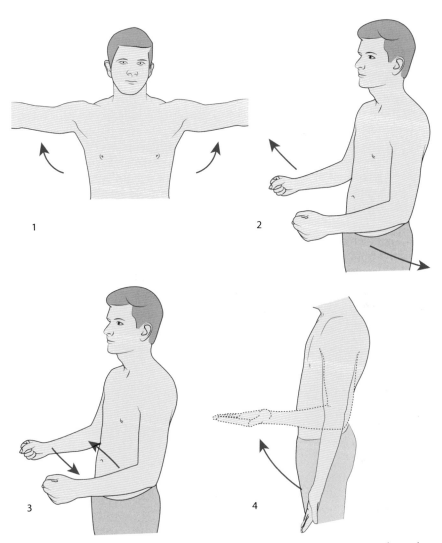

Figure 5.1 What the pain means: 1 resisted abduction; 2 resisted external rotation; 3 resisted internal rotation; 4 resisted supination and flexion of the forearm.

INJECTION TECHNIQUE

Anterior approach (see Figure 5.2)

The patient sits with the arm loosely at the side and externally rotated. Remember that the aim is to inject into the space within the shoulder joint capsule.

Use a 2 ml syringe with a 1 inch (2.5 cm) needle (blue hub) filled with 1 ml steroid solution mixed with 1 ml lidocaine 1% plain. Advance the needle horizontally and in a slightly lateral direction below the acromion process, lateral to the tip of the coracoid process of the scapula and immediately medial to the head of the humerus, all of which are easily palpated. It is especially simple to palpate the head of the humerus anteriorly while passively rotating the humerus internally and externally with the left hand at the bent elbow. Always inject just medially to the head of the humerus; the needle can then only be in the capsule of the shoulder joint. Inject when no resistance is felt to the plunger. Remember that the steroid is injected into the subacromial bursa of the shoulder and not into the glenohumeral joint space, which is relatively narrow and small.

After the injection, ask the patient to repeat the active shoulder joint movements. These movements should now be pain-free because of the local anaesthetic that was mixed with the steroid solution.

Head of humerus   Acromion process   Coracoid process

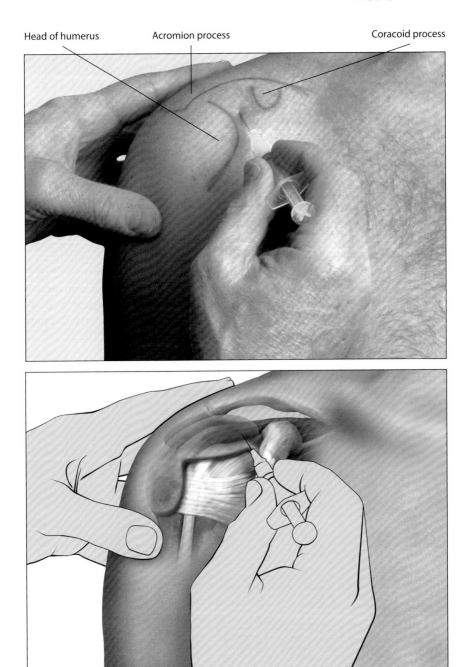

Figure 5.2 Anterior approach.

Lateral (subacromial) approach (see Figure 5.3)

The patient sits with the arm loosely at the side and not rotated. Palpate the most lateral point of the shoulder and make a thumbnail indentation about 0.5 inch (1.3 cm) below the tip of the acromion process. Use 1 ml steroid mixed with 1 ml lidocaine 1% plain in a 2 ml syringe with a 1.5 inch (3.8 cm) needle. The larger needle is advisable as the subcutaneous fat of the upper arm is often quite thick at this point. Advance the needle medially below the acromion process and horizontally and in a slightly posterior direction along the line of the supraspinous fossa. Inject the solution when 1 inch (2.5 cm) of the needle has been inserted.

In subacromial bursitis there is often an effusion, which feels fluctuant to each side of the acromion process. This may be aspirated before injecting the steroid and local anaesthetic mixture. Subacromial bursitis may occur in gout, in Reiter's syndrome following trauma or in rheumatoid arthritis. Sometimes, it may be caused by hydroxyapatite crystals (99% calcium, which forms hydroxyapatite crystals of bone – the mineral of bone). Apart from the presence of an effusion, this condition may be diagnosed by asking the patient to place the arm of the affected side diagonally across the front of the chest. Tapping the point of the elbow will then produce transmitted pain under the acromion process.

The approach to injecting the shoulder joint is more often a personal choice, as the effect of injecting laterally, anteriorly or posteriorly is the same therapeutically for rotator cuff and frozen shoulder problems.

Acromion process

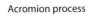

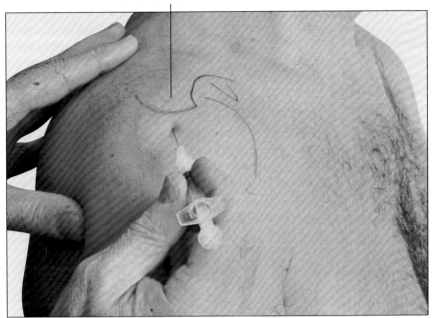

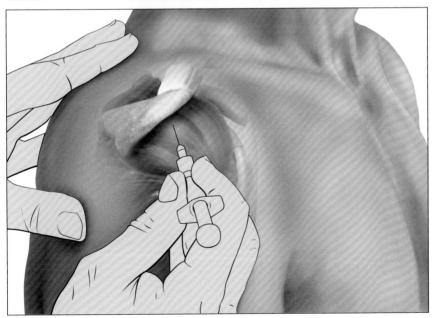

Figure 5.3 Lateral (subacromial) approach.

Posterior approach (see Figure 5.4)

Use 1 ml of steroid mixed with 1 ml lidocaine 1% plain in a 2 ml syringe. Use a 1.5 inch (3.8 cm) needle as, again, the subcutaneous fat over the back is quite thick, especially in an obese patient. The patient sits with the back towards the operator. Palpate the posterior tip of the acromion process with the tip of the thumb. Place the index finger of the same hand on the coracoid process. The imaginary line between the index finger and the thumb marks the track of the needle.

Advance the needle from an entry point approximately 1 inch (2.5 cm) below the tip of the thumb (i.e. below the tip of the acromion and medial to the head of the humerus) about 1 inch (2.5 cm) towards the index finger marking the coracoid process. There will be no resistance to the injection, as the needle point will be in the capsule of the shoulder joint.

This approach is suitable for all rotator cuff lesions and for frozen shoulder.

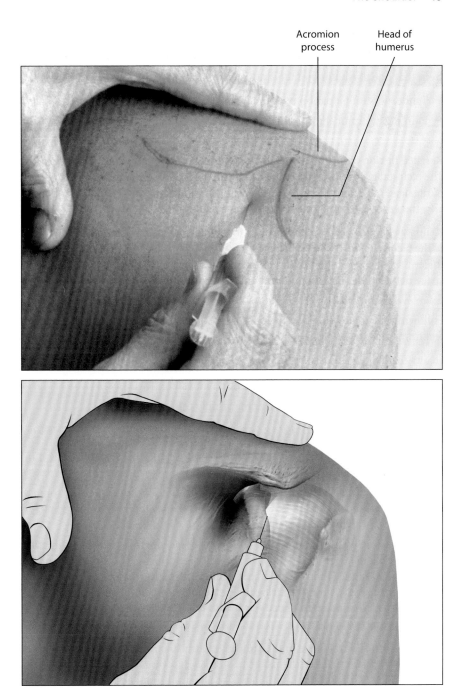

Acromion
process

Head of
humerus

Figure 5.4 Posterior approach.

BICIPITAL TENDINOSIS

The patient complains of pain over the tip of the shoulder. To distinguish this pain from that due to rotator cuff tendinosis, examination of the shoulder will reveal:

- Tenderness on palpation over the bicipital groove.
- Pain at the tip of the shoulder on resisted supination (Yergason's test) of the wrist.

Resisted flexion of the forearm will cause additional pain over the bicipital groove. The bicipital groove (the intertubercular sulcus) is palpable at the anterolateral tip of the head of the humerus. When the subject rotates the arm medially and laterally, the groove becomes more easily identifiable.

It must be emphasised that this condition, which is due to strain of the long head of the biceps tendon, is in fact a tenosynovitis. To cure this condition, the aim is to inject 1 ml of steroid solution mixed with 1 ml lidocaine 1% plain directly into the space between the bicipital tendon and the synovial sheath. Care must be taken not to inject into the substance of the bicipital tendon, which could cause rupture.

Following the injection, if the injection solution is correctly sited, the patient will feel immediate relief of the tenderness and the pain felt on resisted supination.

In any form of tendinosis:

1 Only diagnose if there is pain on resisted movement.
2 Pain in the absence of movement may imply other pathology.

Injection technique (see Figure 5.5)

- Use a 2 ml syringe with a ⅝ inch (1.6 cm) needle. Mix 1 ml of steroid with 1 ml lidocaine 1% plain.
- The patient sits with the affected arm loosely by the side but externally rotated. Make a thumbnail indentation directly over the most tender spot in the bicipital groove, which is easily palpated. This is the site of needle entry.
- Inject just below the skin mark and direct the needle in an upward direction into the bicipital groove. When the needle point enters the substance of the tendon, resistance increases sharply. Maintain gentle pressure on the plunger while at the same time withdrawing the needle slowly until the resistance disappears. At this point the needle is in the synovial sheath, when 2 ml of solution may be injected.

It is rewarding to diagnose and cure this relatively common cause of shoulder pain. In the past, critics of the usage of steroid injections have conjectured that many patients with shoulder pain have not always responded to the injection. It is suggested that, all too often, clinicians have made a diagnosis of bicipital tendinosis without specifically testing and examining the patient, and have vaguely grouped any shoulder pain under the umbrella diagnosis of a rotator cuff lesion. Thus, a more complete differential diagnosis will inevitably lead to a higher success rate in the injection treatment of all these shoulder lesions.

Bicipital groove

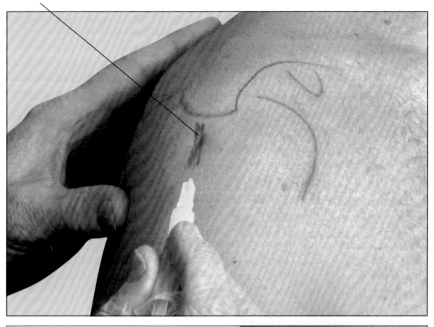

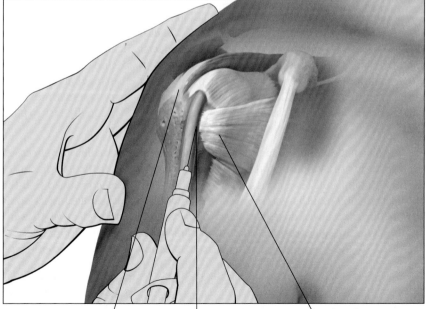

Greater tubercle of   Bicipital tendon   Lesser tubercle of
head of humerus   in its sheath   head of humerus

Figure 5.5 Bicipital tendinosis.

ACROMIOCLAVICULAR JOINT ARTHRITIS

Osteoarthritis of the acromioclavicular joint is a common cause of pain in the patient aged over 50 years. The patient complains of pain directly over the joint, and the diagnosis is confirmed on examination.

- There may be an osteophyte palpable over the joint space itself, which is an obvious indicator that osteoarthritis is present.
- Abduction of the arm from the horizontal to the vertical position will produce pain over the acromioclavicular joint.
- The arm forcefully adducted across the front of the chest under the chin, with the forearm flexed at 90 degrees while protracting the shoulder girdle, causes pain over the acromioclavicular joint.
- Forcefully adducting the arm posteriorly across the back of the chest will produce pain at the limit of adduction.

A diagnostic local injection of local anaesthetic will provide relief of pain. Injection of the acromioclavicular joint with corticosteroid does not alter the natural progression of osteoarthritis but is a valuable procedure for longer-term relief.[2]

Injection technique (see Figure 5.6)

The acromioclavicular joint has a very small joint space that will only accept an injection of between 0.2 and 0.5 ml of fluid. Use a 2 ml syringe with a ⅝ inch (1.6 cm) needle. It is not necessary to mix local anaesthetic. Inject up to 0.5 ml of triamcinolone acetonide. Carefully palpate the joint space and insert the needle either superiorly with a vertical approach, or anteriorly, ensuring that only the tip of the needle enters the joint space. Although the joint space is sometimes difficult to enter on account of the presence of an osteophyte, it is equally easy to push the needle too far and enter the shoulder capsule from above.

Studies reported in 2005 (a meta-analysis, 26 references) revealed the effectiveness, in terms of symptom improvement, of subacromial corticosteroid injections for rotator cuff tendinosis and frozen shoulder. It was concluded that the effect lasted for 9 months, was more effective than NSAIDs and that higher doses were better than lower doses for subacromial corticosteroid injection.[3] A randomised trial in 2005 reported that the shoulder disability questionnaire score improved in those receiving corticosteroid injection, and that physiotherapy improved passive external rotation 6 weeks after treatment.[4] A cost consequences analysis of local corticosteroid shoulder injection and physiotherapy for new episodes of shoulder pain in primary care reported similar clinical outcomes for both treatment groups and that corticosteroid injections were the more cost-effective option.[5] A study in 2006 reported that the prevalence of people consulting for shoulder problems in primary care is substantially lower than community-based estimates. Most referrals occur within three months of initial presentation but only a minority are referred to specialists. It is suggested that, in Oxford, GPs may lack confidence in applying precise diagnosis of shoulder conditions.[6]

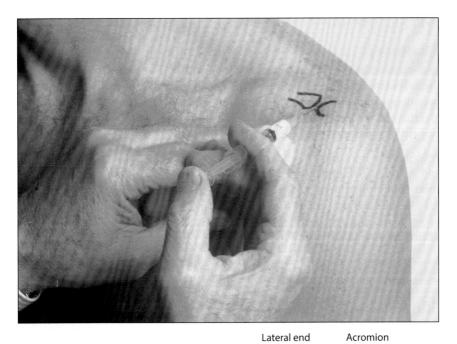

Lateral end
of clavicle

Acromion
process

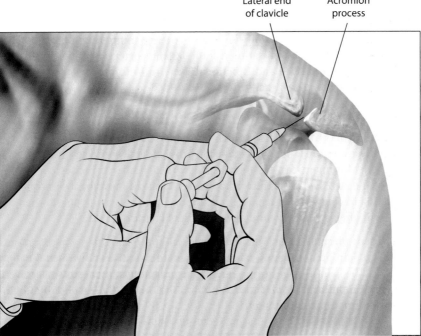

Figure 5.6 Acromioclavicular joint osteoarthritis.

PHYSIOTHERAPY: THE SHOULDER

Summary

Pain-free function of the shoulder is dependent on complex dynamics between the articulations of the scapulothoracic, acromioclavicular, sternoclavicular, glenohumeral and spinal joints. An important aim of physiotherapy treatment is to identify and correct issues in this kinetic chain that are predisposed to the development of shoulder pain.

Poor posture is a common underlying issue and is typified by the slumped spine and protracted shoulders experienced when sitting at a computer. Maintaining good spinal alignment with the shoulders relaxed and slightly retracted will reduce stress on the spinal and shoulder joints. This good posture should also be maintained during normal daily activities. Detailed ergonomic and lifestyle advice can be given as part of a physiotherapy programme.

There are specific areas of advice and rehabilitation pertinent to the injections described in this book.

Shoulder impingement

In the absence of an acute cuff tear, physiotherapy and injection remain first-line treatment in subacromial impingement syndrome. The pain relief provided by corticosteroid injection can provide a window of opportunity for rehabilitation. This would include strengthening the rotator cuff and improving soft tissue flexibility with exercise and mobilisation techniques and correction of postural issues with strapping and advice and functional exercise to improve scapulothoracic control during normal daily activity.

'Frozen' shoulder/shoulder capsulitis

Physiotherapy has a limited role when constant or night pain is the dominant issue. In these circumstances, injection can provide rapid short- to medium-term pain relief. Movement can be encouraged with pendular exercises, where the weight of the arm swings within the pain-free range of movement. Prescription of analgesia to control nocturnal pain is important in this acute phase when the patient will often struggle to find any position of comfort.

If the patient presents in the 'thawing stage' of frozen shoulder, where stiffness rather than pain predominates, manual therapy to mobilise and stretch the joint capsule can be helpful in restoring range. The patient usually needs to persevere with several months of regular stretching into shoulder elevation and rotation to restore full functional movement.

Acromioclavicular joint arthritis

Passive joint mobilisation can help in restoring range of movement to the acromioclavicular and sternoclavicular joints. Advice on establishing good shoulder posture and avoiding repeated horizontal shoulder adduction reduces compression through the acromioclavicular joint and so reduces pain.

REFERENCES

1   Akgun K *et al* (2004) Is local subacromial corticosteroid injection beneficial in subacromial impingement syndrome? *Clin Rheumatol.* **23** (6): 496–500.

2   Buttaci CJ *et al* (2004) Osteoarthritis of the acromioclavicular joint: a review of anatomy, biomechanics, diagnosis and treatment. Review [24 references]. *Am J Phys Med Rehabil.* **83** (10): 791–797.

3   Arroll B and Goodyear-Smith F (2005) Corticosteroid injections for painful shoulder: a meta-analysis. *Br J Gen Pract.* **55**: 224–228.

4   Ryans I *et al* (2005) A randomised controlled trial of intra-articular triamcinolone and/or physiotherapy in shoulder capsulitis. *Rheumatol.* **44**: 529–535.

5   James M *et al* (2005) A cost analysis of local corticosteroid injection and physiotherapy for the treatment of new episodes of unilateral shoulder pain in primary care. *Rheumatol.* **44** (11): 1447–1451.

6   Linsell L *et al* (2006) Prevalence and incidence of adults consulting for shoulder conditions in UK primary care: patterns of referral and diagnosis. *Rheumatol.* **45** (2): 215–221.

7   Uppal HS *et al* (2015). Frozen shoulder: a systematic review of therapeutic options. *World J Orthop.* **6** (2): 263–268.

8   Bunker TD and Anthony PP (1995) The pathology of frozen shoulder. A Dupuytren-like disease. *J Bone Joint Surg Br.* **77**: 677–683.

CHAPTER 6

The wrist and hand

INCIDENCE

Soft tissue lesions commonly occur in the wrist joint, hand and fingers. Rheumatoid arthritis (RA) and other arthropathies predispose to some of these problems. Osteoarthritis is about four times more common than RA. Primary osteoarthritis runs in families as an autosomal dominant trait. The most familiar pattern affects the terminal interphalangeal joints, producing Heberden's nodes, as well as affecting the carpometacarpal joint of the thumb. In osteoarthritis of the other joints, genetic influences are less obvious. Secondary arthritis may follow sporting activities and trauma that produce recurrent traumatic synovitis.

COMMON PROBLEMS TREATED WITH STEROID INJECTIONS

- *Osteoarthritis.* Affecting the first carpometacarpal joint (thumb).
- *Rheumatoid arthritis.* Acute exacerbations of the interphalangeal or carpometacarpal joints.
- *Carpal tunnel syndrome.* This is due to median nerve compression (nerve entrapment) at the wrist. This condition may be predisposed by conditions that cause weight increase, such as obesity, myxoedema, acromegaly, pregnancy, RA, collagen disorders, osteoarthritis and previous trauma affecting the bones of the wrist joint. The condition occurs more frequently in females and in those taking the oral contraceptive pill.
- *Tenosynovitis of the thumb (de Quervain's disease).* The extensor pollicis brevis and the abductor pollicis longus tendons are particularly prone to inflammation following occupational trauma or repetitive stress.
- *Trigger finger.* This condition may be idiopathic, but occurs more commonly in RA (it may be an early or late manifestation). It may affect any of the flexor tendon synovial sheaths in the palm, including the thumb.

THE FIRST CARPOMETACARPAL JOINT

The first carpometacarpal joint is one of the few joints affected by osteoarthritis in which the response to steroid injection is rewarding (the other joint responding well to steroid injection is the acromioclavicular joint). Commonly described as 'washerwomen's thumb', this type of osteoarthritis follows the repetitive chores undertaken in the course of domestic work.

Presentation and diagnosis

The patient commonly complains of aching around the joint, and examination reveals pain on passive backward movement of the thumb in extension. Often osteophytes are present, noted on radiographic examination of the joint. These may render injection into the small joint space difficult.

Functional anatomy

This joint is the articulation of the first metacarpal with the trapezium bone of the wrist. Extension and abduction of the thumb causes pain and there is deep tenderness in the 'anatomical snuffbox' at the joint line, which is more easily palpable when the subject flexes and tucks the thumb into the palm. The joint space, although small, will accept an injection of about 0.5 ml of steroid solution.

Injection technique (see Figure 6.1)

The patient tucks the thumb as far into the palm as possible and holds it there with the index and middle fingers. Palpate the joint line dorsally and then inject from the lateral aspect, taking care to avoid the abductor pollicis tendon as it marks the border of the snuffbox. Use a small ⅝ inch (1.6 cm) needle and inject up to 0.5 ml triamcinolone acetonide. No lidocaine is required, although some doctors prefer to use an equal quantity of lidocaine 1% plain.

Trapezium   Base of first metacarpal

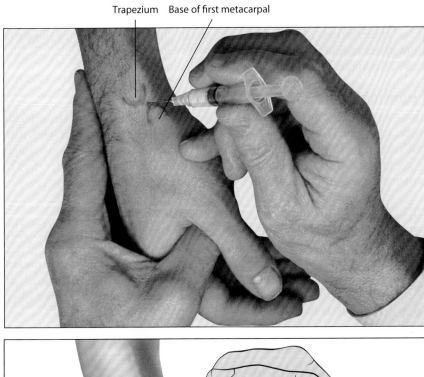

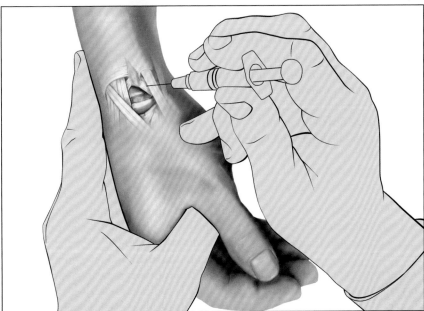

Figure 6.1 The first carpometacarpal joint.

METACARPAL AND INTERPHALANGEAL JOINTS

Acute exacerbations of RA affecting the small joints of the hands often benefit from direct injection of steroids, such as triamcinolone acetonide, into the joint space or into the surrounding inflamed synovium and capsule.

Functional anatomy

These are simple joints, but it must be remembered that the joint space of the metacarpal joint is distal to the knuckle on palpation and is a condylar joint, with one palmar and two collateral ligaments. The interphalangeal joints are simple hinge joints, each with a palmar and two collateral ligaments. It is important to remember the neurovascular bundle at the side of each joint when injecting.

Injection technique

Palpate the joint line often by applying some gentle traction to open up the joint space before injecting 0.25–0.5 ml triamcinolone acetonide anterolaterally into the joint space. As the joint spaces are so small, it is not necessary to mix the steroid with lidocaine unless the joints are very tender on palpation. Injection of two or three of these joints at a time is appropriate and, often, a long-lasting remission of up to 6 months is attained.[1]

CARPAL TUNNEL SYNDROME

Presentation and diagnosis

This is probably the most common nerve entrapment disorder, affecting women more commonly than men. It is caused by compression of the median nerve as it enters the palm posterior to the flexor retinaculum. The typical syndrome presents as pain radiating up the arm from the wrist, with paraesthesia affecting the median nerve distribution in the palm, namely the thumb, index and predominantly the middle finger and lateral half of the ring finger; symptoms can paroxysmally affect the patient in the night and be relieved on getting up and moving the arm and hand around. If left untreated, the condition may deteriorate and produce muscle wasting in the thenar eminence of the palm.

The middle finger is often the first and the worst finger to be affected by the paraesthesia. Occasionally the patient complains of paraesthesia affecting all the fingers of the hand, and this produces a diagnostic problem for the clinician. This may be due to a total entrapment of both the ulnar and median nerves. It is known that there may be anatomical connections between the ulnar and median nerves to account for this, and if the history is typical as described, a diagnosis of carpal tunnel syndrome may still confidently be made even though the patient complains of paraesthesia in all the fingers.

As described earlier, it is important to recognise and treat any of the predisposing or concomitant disorders in order to ensure a lasting recovery.

Tinel's test

This is a reliable diagnostic test. Percuss lightly over the flexor retinaculum with a tendon hammer, particularly between the palmaris longus tendon and the flexor carpi radialis tendons. The test is positive if the patient describes a tingling sensation in the median nerve distribution.

Phelan's test

This is another useful confirmatory test. Hold the wrist in acute flexion for up to 1 minute; this usually reproduces the pain and typical paraesthesia.

Diagnosis may be confirmed by electromyography, and this further test is recommended in cases of doubt. It is often necessary to exclude causes of paraesthesia in the hand or pain in the arm arising from the cervical spine, such as cervical disc lesions or spondylosis causing C5 or C6 nerve entrapments.

Functional anatomy

The median nerve lies posterior to the palmaris longus tendon at the wrist, and it enters the palm deep to the flexor retinaculum. The latter is a dense fibrous band covering the proximal one-third of the palm, into which the palmaris longus tendon is inserted. The palmaris longus tendon is the most central and superficial tendon, which is prominent when the wrist is flexed against resistance. Consequently, it is important to identify the palmaris longus tendon as this enables the operator to know the exact position of the median nerve. Approximately 13% of people do not possess a palmaris longus, in which case the median nerve is then identified as lying between the tendons of the flexor digitorum superficialis and the flexor carpi radialis. On entering the palm, the median nerve then lies in the carpal tunnel, where it divides into its digital branches.

Injection technique (see Figure 6.2)

Treatment of a mild carpal tunnel syndrome may, initially, be simple weight reduction advice together with a daily diuretic tablet, such as hydrochlorothiazide or cyclopenthiazide. Night splints may also help and may be the preferred management in early pregnancy. It is unwise to inject steroids in the first 16–18 weeks of pregnancy. If these simple measures are not successful, steroid injection is advisable and will be helpful in over 60% of cases. If there is no response to steroid injection (after two or three successive injections) or, very importantly, if there is evidence of median nerve damage, such as thenar eminence muscle wasting, it is wise to refer for surgical decompression.

The patient sits facing the operator, with the palm of the affected hand facing upwards and resting on a firm surface. By flexing the wrist against resistance, the palmaris longus tendon is clearly seen. Make a thumbnail indentation or skin mark on the radial side of the tendon precisely at the distal crease of the wrist; this is the best injection site. As in all these procedures, it is kinder to the patient to inject, where possible, through a skin crease as this ensures less pain. If you cannot demonstrate the palmaris tendon, which is absent in 13% of patients, palpate the gap between the tendons of the flexor digitorum superficialis and the flexor carpi radialis and then mark the skin at the distal crease. Ensure that you avoid any surface veins.

Use 1 ml of steroid, for example, triamcinolone acetonide alone, in a 2 ml syringe. Use a 1 inch (2.5 cm) needle. No local anaesthetic is added, because its effect may cause an uncomfortable numbness in the fingers and palm in the median nerve distribution, lasting for several hours. The symptoms of carpal tunnel syndrome are very unpleasant for many patients, so reproducing these symptoms for several hours will produce much discomfort, not to mention causing some unpopularity for the doctor!

With the wrist now straight, advance the needle almost to the hilt, pointing distally and at an angle of 45 degrees. This ensures that the steroid solution is deposited in the carpal tunnel immediately behind the flexor retinaculum. At this moment, always ask the patient if this is comfortable and ensure that no pain is felt. Inadvertent needling of a digital branch of the median nerve will cause pain in the palm that can be referred along a finger. If this should occur, just withdraw the needle slightly before injecting. Aspirate to exclude any intravascular injection. You should then be able to inject the steroid easily, with little resistance to the plunger. Inject slowly, as this will ensure the least pain or discomfort produced by the injection.

The median nerve lies posterior to the palmaris longus tendon. If the needle insertion causes immediate paraesthesia, indicating that the needle has entered the substance of the median nerve, withdraw the needle slightly and reinsert it laterally. This will ensure that no damage is caused to the nerve itself.

Always remember to remind the patient that some acute pain may be experienced for up to 48 hours after the injection. Advise that simple analgesia is effective, and instruct the patient to rest the arm for 24–48 hours after the injection.

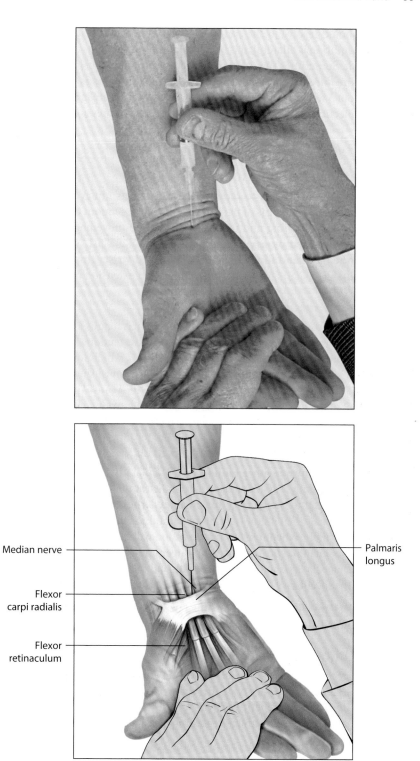

Median nerve

Palmaris longus

Flexor carpi radialis

Flexor retinaculum

Figure 6.2 Carpal tunnel syndrome.

Symptoms should resolve in the course of a few days, and reassurance is important. If the condition is bilateral, it is better to inject one side initially and await the clinical result. Sometimes the other side improves spontaneously and no further treatment is required. Where no improvement in symptoms is noted, a second injection about 3 weeks later is justified. However, where there is no improvement after three injections, it is wise to refer for surgical decompression.[2]

DE QUERVAIN'S TENOSYNOVITIS

Presentation and diagnosis

This condition is usually due to repetitive strain, sports injury or occupational hazard. The patient complains of pain in the line of the tendon. On examination, there may be some swelling and crepitus palpated on movement of the thumb. Diagnosis is confirmed by asking the patient to make a fist while flexing the thumb into the palm and ulnar-deviating the flexed wrist. This reproduces the pain. The pain also occurs on abduction and resisted extension of the thumb.

Functional anatomy

De Quervain's tenosynovitis affects the abductor pollicis longus and extensor pollicis brevis tendons, which have become inflamed. These tendons fuse as they cross the radial styloid and form a common synovial sheath, which forms the anterior border of the 'snuffbox'. The tendons are lined with a synovial sheath, and in tenosynovitis, the synovial surfaces become roughened, which causes pain and crepitus on movement of the tendon. In injecting, the aim is to introduce the steroid mixed with local anaesthetic into the space between the tendon and the sheath.

Injection technique (see Figure 6.3)

Use 1 ml of steroid mixed with 1 ml lidocaine 1% plain in a 2 ml syringe, using a ⅝ inch (1.6 cm) (number 20, 25 gauge) needle. Insert the needle along the line of the tendon just distal to the point of maximal tenderness, advancing it proximally into the substance of the tendon (it is more painful for the patient if this injection is introduced distally), when resistance to injection will be felt. Slowly withdraw the needle, while maintaining pressure on the plunger until the resistance disappears. At this point, the needle tip is in the tendon sheath and the whole 2 ml of solution may be injected. The sheath may visibly expand along its course as the solution is injected.

One may select any of the steroids for this purpose. Relief of pain is usually dramatic and immediate.

Post-injection advice

It is wise to recommend a period of rest of the affected part for a few days and avoidance of painful movements or the tasks that initially caused the problem. Recurrences indicate that repetitive strain, possibly as a result of faulty technique, is the cause, and appropriate advice regarding occupation should be sought.

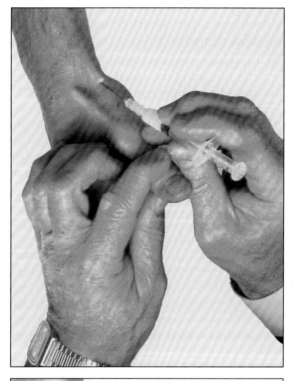

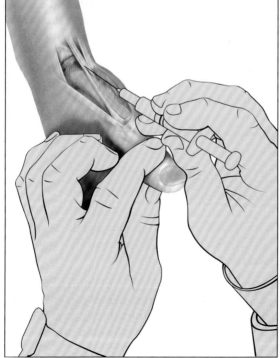

Figure 6.3 De Quervain's tenosynovitis.

TRIGGER FINGER

Presentation and diagnosis

Trigger finger may be idiopathic but it is common in early and late RA and affects any or all of the flexor tendons of the fingers in the palm. A tender nodule in the palm is usually palpated over the line of the flexor tendon just proximal to the metacarpophalangeal joint crease. Injection will be into the tendon sheath and not into this nodule. The patient complains of an uncomfortable locking of the affected finger spontaneously occurring in flexion; only with difficulty can the finger be released by manipulating or forcefully extending the affected joint. Naturally this condition is an occupational hazard for anyone undertaking machine or intricate work involving the hands and fingers.

Functional anatomy

This condition is a tenosynovitis affecting any of the flexor tendons (superficial and deep) in the palm. These tendons are enveloped by synovial sheaths as they traverse the carpal tunnel. They extend for about 1 inch (2.5 cm) above the flexor retinaculum to about halfway along each metacarpal, except for the little finger, in which the sheath is continuous and extends to the terminal phalanx, and the thumb (flexor pollicis longus), where the sheath is continuous to the tip of the finger. The fibrous synovial sheaths of the terminal parts of the tendons are thinner over the joints.

Injection technique (see Figure 6.4)

Use 1 ml steroid mixed with 1 ml lidocaine 1% plain in a 2 ml syringe with a ⅝ inch (1.6 cm) needle. Insert the needle over the crease overlying the metacarpophalangeal joint and advance it proximally into the flexor tendon. Ask the patient to flex that finger, which will move the needle, confirming that the needle point is in the tendon. Resistance to the plunger will be experienced. Slowly withdraw the needle while maintaining pressure on the plunger until resistance to injection disappears, when the contents may easily be injected into the tendon sheath. A slow injection of the solution will expand the part of the tendon sheath proximal to the injection, a confirmatory sign that the steroid is in the correct place.

It is important to emphasise that one should never attempt to inject steroid into the substance of a tendon. As stated previously, these injections should be easy with no force required, and the solution should just glide in.

Trigger fingers respond well to steroid injection, but do recur and may be injected two to three times in a year, if clinically required. However, further recurrences may need a surgical release.[3]

Image guidance using ultrasound may assist in confirming the diagnosis of focal tenosynovitis, and dynamic examination allows correlation of symptoms and findings to confirm the diagnosis. A targeted injection to the tendon sheath or 'seed ganglion', frequently encountered as the focal cause of triggering, may be helpful.

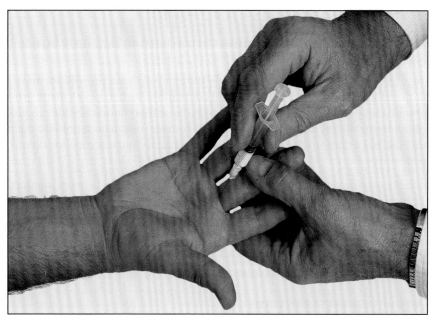

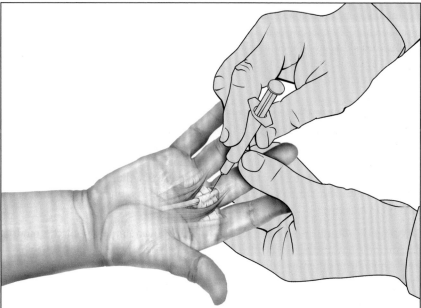

Figure 6.4 Trigger finger.

PHYSIOTHERAPY: WRIST AND HAND

First carpometacarpal, metacarpal and interphalangeal joint osteoarthritis

The effects of arthritis in the small joints of the hand can have a significant impact on the tasks of daily life. Simple aids and adaptations such as plastic hand grips around pens, jars and bottles can make everyday activity easier. A wide range of splints are available, ranging from 'over-the-counter' neoprene splints for night time use, to custom-made moulded orthoses, which facilitate occupational tasks.

Daily exercises to maintain range of movement can be supplemented by the patient carrying out their own joint mobilisations. These can be more comfortably performed with the hand in warm water. Increasing the strength of the thenar, hypothenar and intrinsic hand muscles improves the stability of the small hand joints during normal daily use.

Topical NSAIDs have been shown to be effective in hand osteoarthritis and can be useful adjuncts to simple analgesia.

Carpal tunnel syndrome

Although physiotherapy can be used to treat carpal tunnel syndrome, the results are inconsistent and slow. The positive effect of corticosteroid injection can be supplemented by exercises and soft tissue techniques to ensure that the normal gliding and shearing movement of the median nerve within the carpal tunnel is restored and maintained. A wrist splint can ease nocturnal symptoms in acute or chronic situations.

De Quervain's tenosynovitis

Physiotherapy can be considered if injection is preferably avoided (e.g. in breast-feeding women, where there is increased risk of depigmentation/fat atrophy/tendon rupture, or in recurrent cases, if there has been partial response to injection). Alternatives to injection include the use of a thumb splint or strapping to support and rest the inflamed structures, ice packs, ultrasound and specific soft tissue massage.

Early gentle thumb movement will maintain movement between the tendon, sheath and surrounding tissue interfaces, but should be performed within a pain-free range. Strengthening surrounding muscles, including eccentric activity of the extensor carpi ulnaris, aims to reduce the stress through the affected tendons.

Tenosynovitis usually occurs secondary to overuse, so advice on good working practices forms an important part of sustaining improvement and preventing recurrence.

Trigger finger

The curative effect of most corticosteroid injections means that physiotherapy is rarely needed for trigger finger or thumb. In the early stages, strapping or splinting of the affected finger into extension will allow the flexor tendon to rest and may abolish the trigger should injection need to be avoided.

REFERENCES

1 Raman J (2005) Intra-articular corticosteroid injection for first carpometacarpal osteoarthritis. *J Rheumatol.* **32**: 1305–1306.

2 Agarwal V *et al* (2005) A prospective study of the long-term efficacy of local methyl prednisolone acetate injection in the management of mild carpal tunnel syndrome. *Rheumatol.* **44** (5): 647–650.

3 Nimigan A *et al* (2006) Steroid injections in the management of trigger fingers. *Am J Phys Med Rehabil.* **85** (1): 36–43.

CHAPTER 7

The elbow

INTRODUCTION

Perhaps the most common soft tissue lesions are those affecting the extensor and flexor insertions at the elbow, as in tennis and golfer's elbow, so called because the bad tennis forearm drive or the bad golf swing reputedly causes these conditions. In these lesions, the tendon substance (tenoperiosteal junction), which has no synovial sheath, itself becomes inflamed or degenerative and is a tendinopathy rather than an inflammatory tenosynovitis (in which the tendon synovial sheath becomes inflamed).

TENNIS ELBOW

Acute tennis elbow is common in young- to middle-aged patients owing to strain of the extensor tendons of the forearm. Also known as lateral epicondylitis, it is a strain occurring at the tenoperiosteal insertion into the extensor epicondyle of the humerus. It is often caused by repetitive movements at work, such as screw-driving or polishing. A defective backhand or forehand drive at tennis, squash or badminton is often a causative factor.

Very rarely, a bony secondary deposit may cause pain and tenderness on palpation, which is not reproduced by resisted extension of the wrist. If in doubt, obtain radiographs of the elbow joint before injecting steroids.

Ultrasound or MRI may be helpful in atypical or refractory cases to allow confirmation of diagnosis and to exclude alternative pathology.

Presentation and diagnosis

On palpation, there is exquisite pain and localised tenderness over the lateral epicondyle of the humerus. This pain may be reproduced by asking the patient to extend the hand at the wrist (dorsiflexion) against resistance. All other movements at the elbow are normal.

Functional anatomy

The common insertion of the extensor muscles of the forearm and the hand is the lateral epicondyle of the humerus. These muscles are essentially the brachioradialis, extensor carpi radialis, extensor carpi ulnaris and digitorum muscles. Strain of any of these muscles at their insertion will cause a tendinosis at this site, which will produce an easily localised point of acute tenderness. Asking the patient to extend the wrist against resistance enables the operator to pinpoint the lesion accurately.

Injection technique (see Figure 7.1)

Use 1 ml of steroid in a 2 ml syringe with a ⅝ inch (1.6 cm) needle. Personal choice will dictate whether or not to mix the steroid with local anaesthetic. It is important to remember that local anaesthetic, such as lidocaine, is so effective that it will prevent the discovery of all the tender points of the lesion. Using steroid alone is more painful for the patient, but the overall success of the injection is higher because the operator will be able to detect all the painful or tender parts

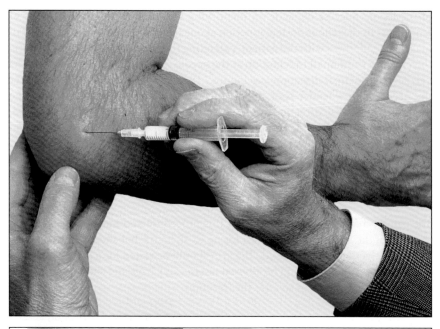

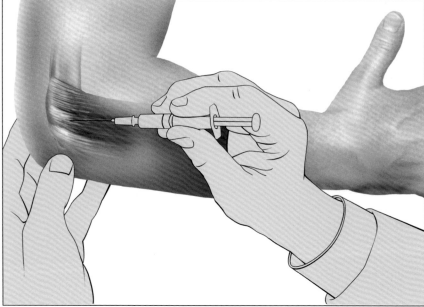

Figure 7.1 Tennis elbow.

of the lesion. Success depends on identifying and infiltrating all the points of tenderness in the tenoperiosteal junction at one injection. First locate the point of maximal tenderness with the patient, extending the hand against your resistance; then make a thumbnail indentation at the needle entry point. After inserting the needle in a proximal direction (*see* Figure 7.1), ask the patient each time whether the needle is in a tender spot, subcutaneously moving the needle around the lesion in a clockwise direction and in a fan shape after the initial skin puncture, and ensuring that all tender points are injected accurately with about 0.1–0.2 ml of steroid each time, delivering in all up to 1 ml of steroid.

Using this technique of infiltrating all the tender parts of the tendinosis lesion, one can be more assured of complete success in treating tennis and golfer's elbow, and also in lessening the frequently reported recurrences.

The patient may sit or lie down during this procedure and must be warned that the pain of the injection may persist for up to 48 hours, but should then subside. Simple analgesia may be advised. The arm should be rested for a day or two after the injection. Patients should be advised not to carry bags and shopping with the affected arm for a week or so after the injection.

GOLFER'S ELBOW

This condition mirrors the lesion of tennis elbow, occurring in the origin of the forearm flexor muscles at the medial epicondyle of the humerus. Also known as medial epicondylitis, it may be due to the golf player's faulty backswing and to other repetitive movements affecting the flexor muscle group.

Presentation and diagnosis

The patient complains of acute tenderness on a spot over the medial epicondyle, which is easily reproduced at this site by asking the patient to flex the hand at the wrist against resistance.

Functional anatomy

The common tendon insertion of the muscles of the flexor group at the medial epicondyle is affected. They are the flexor carpi radialis, digitorum superficialis, flexor carpi ulnaris and palmaris longus. As in tennis elbow, the lesion is localised to the tenoperiosteal junction. It is important to recall that the ulnar nerve is in close proximity in the canal posterior to the medial epicondyle, and may be easily punctured by the injecting needle. Prior to the injection, when the needle is *in situ*, the doctor should confirm that no paraesthesiae are felt in the ulnar distribution (i.e. in the little finger and the ulnar side of the ring finger).

Injection technique (see Figure 7.2)

The patient sits with his back to the operator or lies on a couch with the fore-arm of the affected side behind the back and the dorsum of the hand resting on the buttock. The tender spot in the medial epicondyle is identified by asking the patient to flex the hand against resistance. Mark the spot with a thumbnail inden-tation as the site of needle entry.

Use 1 ml of steroid in a 2 ml syringe with a ⅝ inch (1.6 cm) needle and proceed to infiltrate all the tender spots of the lesion precisely as described earlier for treat-ing tennis elbow.

POST-INJECTION ADVICE

Avoid painful movements for the next few days after the injection. Remember that there may be 'after pain' for up to 48 hours, after which the condition is expected to improve. Simple analgesic tablets may be all that are required for a day or so. Repeat injections may be given at 3- or 4-weekly intervals, up to a total of three injections in 12 months, if necessary.

LIPODYSTROPHY

Remember that both tennis and golfer's elbow are superficial lesions and the injection must be made deeply into the fibrous substance of the tenoperiosteal junction. This effectively means that the needle point may well touch the perios-teum. If this is not ensured, it is all too easy to inject steroid into the subcutane-ous fat, in which case dimpling of the skin due to fat dissolution may occur. It is always wise when injecting these lesions to warn the patient beforehand of this possibility in order to minimise any future complaint of negligence. The more potent intra-articular steroids have the reputation of causing lipodystrophy, but any steroid preparation injected into the subcutaneous fat layer may produce it.

Ultrasound-guided injections may be helpful, and dry needling at the same pro-cedure may also be helpful. Variable evidence with regard to injecting protein rich plasma is available in the literature, and this may be an option to consider.

PHYSIOTHERAPY: TENNIS AND GOLFER'S ELBOW

In common with other degenerative tendinopathies, the use of corticoste-roid injection is recognised as providing effective but short-term pain relief. Prevention of chronicity or recurrence relies on addressing the causative factors with a combination of advice and/or physiotherapy.

Reducing mechanical load through the painful tendon is key in easing the acute stage of tennis and golfer's elbow, and may involve stopping all pain-provoking activity for a short period. Pain-relieving modalities include use of simple oral or topical analgesia/NSAIDs, ice packs, acupuncture and soft tissue massage.

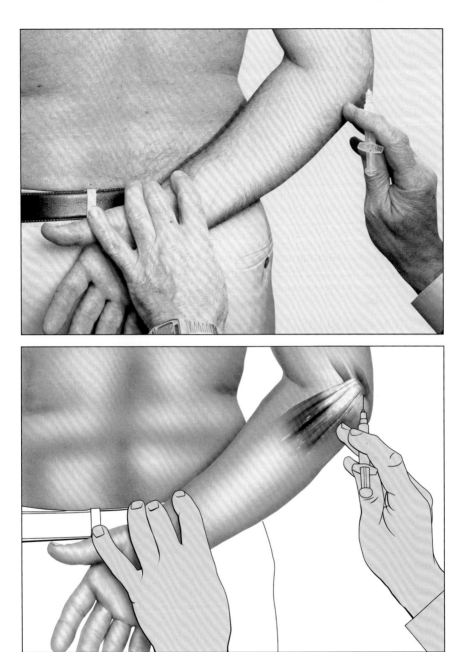

Figure 7.2 Golfer's elbow.

Long-term adoption of good working habits can include reducing the weight or frequency of the use of heavy tools and by carrying with the elbow flexed rather than extended. Repetitive activity at low load such as that involved in keyboard use is also a risk factor. Improvement in working posture can be achieved by using a combination of chair, desk and display screen, which maintains the spine and upper limbs in a neutral position. Detailed information is freely available on the internet (e.g. http://www.nhs.uk/Livewell/workplacehealth/Pages/howtositcorrectly.aspx).

Further modification of the tendon load can be supplemented in cases of tennis elbow by use of an elbow brace.

Muscle weakness and poor soft tissue flexibility reduce the ability of a tendon to withstand load effectively. Exercises to improve the strength of the wrist extensors can be added early if they are carried out in a pain-free manner with the elbow flexed and the wrist in mid position. As improvement occurs, the programme progresses to incorporating exercise at higher speed, frequency and resistance. Soft tissue deficits can be improved with soft tissue mobilisation such as deep friction massage, Mills manipulation, joint mobilisation and stretching exercises.

OLECRANON BURSITIS (SEE FIGURE 7.3)

This condition is one of several painful bursa problems commonly occurring in general practice. It may occur following repeated minor trauma, and is also known as 'student's elbow'. It may also occur in gout and should be investigated when there is no other obvious cause. In rheumatoid disease, nodules may be palpable in this bursa. In gout, tophi may be present.

The synovial tissue behind the elbow joint and the olecranon process is quite profuse and lax and, commonly, a bursa filled with clear, yellow, viscous effusion appears. The swelling appears and often enlarges in size, and can be quite tense and fluctuant on palpation. Sometimes the bursa is reddened with acute sepsis, which may require antibiotic therapy. There is, however, more often no obvious infection, and aspiration is a simple matter. A 1.5 inch (3.8 cm) needle is inserted into the bursa and the fluid aspirated using a 10 ml syringe. Occasionally, these bursae may be loculated, and it is necessary to move the needle point around within the bursa to completely evacuate the serous contents.

Microscopy may reveal polymorphonuclear leucocytes, in infection, or urate crystals, in gout. A firm Tubigrip bandage should be applied afterwards to prevent the bursa refilling. Repeated aspiration may be necessary. In frequent recurrences, it is helpful to inject these with 1 ml of steroid after aspiration, with a fair chance of preventing the recurrence of the condition.

Following injection and aspiration, apply a firm elastic or double Tubigrip support around the elbow. This may help prevent the bursa refilling with fluid.

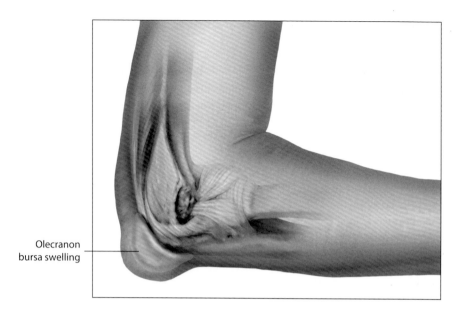

Olecranon
bursa swelling

Figure 7.3 Olecranon bursitis.

ELBOW JOINT (SEE FIGURE 7.4)

Presentation

Painful elbow occurs in exacerbations of arthritis and post-traumatic synovitis (e.g. following the unaccustomed carrying of heavy objects such as luggage with the arm extended). All movements of flexion, pronation and supination aggravate the pain.

Functional anatomy

The elbow joint comprises the trochlea of the humerus, articulating with the trochlear notch of the ulna (olecranon), in addition to the articulation of the radial head with the lower end of the humerus (the capitulum). The synovial membrane is extensive and, together with extrasynovial fat, forms a soft palpable pad, anteriorly. The easiest way to inject the joint is by palpating anterolaterally into this soft pad, using the finger to determine the bone edges between the lateral epicondyle of the humerus, the olecranon process and the head of the radius. A triangle is formed, the centre of which is the best point for needle insertion. Gentle passive movement of the forearm and the radial head by pronating and supinating reveals the joint space outline and facilitates the injection.

Injection technique

Sit the patient, with the forearm at an angle of 90 degrees resting on the examination couch or a table. Make a thumbnail imprint at the point of injection, as earlier, resting the examining finger on an alcohol swab. Insert the needle in an anterolateral direction 1–2 cm and slowly inject a solution of steroid, such as 1 ml triamcinolone acetonide mixed with 1–3 ml lidocaine 1% plain, using a blue hub 1 inch (2.5 cm) needle. The injection should be quite easy and free. If resistance to injection is noticed, then gently move the needle slightly until completion is easy.

PHYSIOTHERAPY: ELBOW JOINT

Restoration of functional movement following injection can be encouraged with regular movement in a pain-free range repeated every few hours. The initial emphasis should be on improving elbow flexion, as this is vital in many everyday activities, such as eating and personal hygiene.

Patients with persistent stiffness or weakness, which fails to improve with simple exercises, should be referred for early physiotherapy.

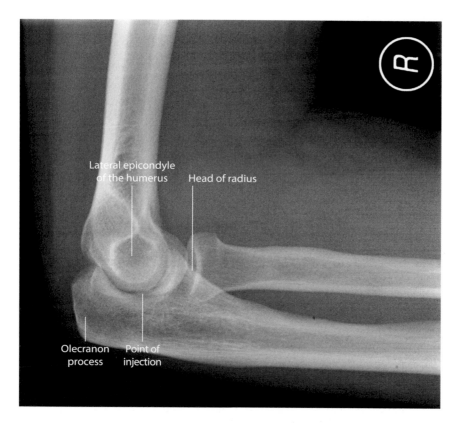

Figure 7.4 Lateral radiograph, right elbow.

Chapter 8

Conditions around the hip and thigh

THE HIP

Steroid injections into the hip joint are no longer commonly performed. The procedure is more complicated than for other intra-articular injections, and it is not advisable for general practitioners to undertake such injections. Moreover, the management of osteoarthritis of the hip joint has radically changed in the last few years due to the success of hip replacement operations and the marked improvement of the hip prostheses that are now fitted. However, there are several conditions that are easily treated in the practice.

TROCHANTERIC BURSITIS

This may occur in rheumatoid arthritis or following minor trauma. The patient complains of pain around the hip. On further enquiry, it is apparent that the pain is felt laterally over the greater trochanter of the femur, worse when lying on the affected side in bed at night. There is localised tenderness around the greater trochanter, and there may be fullness on palpation if there is fluid in the bursa of gluteus medius or minimus.

Recent evidence confirms that this commonly encountered diagnosis related to underlying tendinosis of the abductor tendons is rarely related to an inflammatory aetiology, suggesting the previous diagnosis of 'trochanteric bursitis' is a misnomer.

Consensus opinions of orthopaedic physicians and sports medicine specialists have recently suggested that trochanteric bursitis should be better known as greater trochanter pain syndrome (GTPS).[1]

It is postulated that the significant short-term superiority of a single corticosteroid injection over home training and shockwave therapy declines after 1 month. This condition is a painful overuse syndrome of the hip in adults engaging in recreational sports activities. The anatomical relationship between three bursae, the hip adductor–external rotator muscles, the greater trochanter and the overlying iliotibial tract (band), may predispose this area to biomechanical irritation. Magnetic resonance imaging studies have shown abnormalities that appear to better correlate with the GTPS than any other bursal lesion. These studies showed swellings of the trochanteric bursa to be uncommon – hence the suggestion to label all these conditions of pain around the lateral hip joint as GTPS.

Injection technique (see Figure 8.1)

The patient lies on the couch with the affected side uppermost and the hip flexed. At the most tender spot over the trochanter, perpendicularly insert a 1 inch (2.5 cm) needle attached to a 10 ml syringe until the bone is reached. Withdraw the needle slightly and aspirate the clear yellow fluid. Then, leaving the needle *in situ*, change the syringe so that 1 ml of steroid may be injected into the bursa and the tough fibrous insertion of the gluteal fascia.

Beware that the bursa in some patients may be beyond the reach of a short standard needle. Depending upon body habitus, a longer 'spinal type needle' maybe required.

If the injection fails to result in symptomatic relief, even in the short term, consider an ultrasound-guided injection to allow definitive placement of steroid.

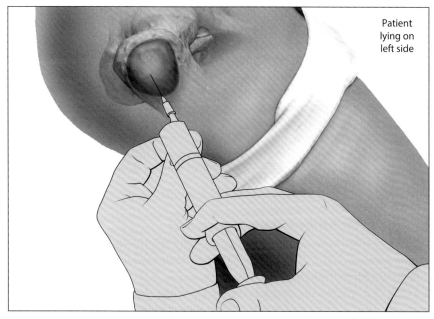

Patient lying on left side

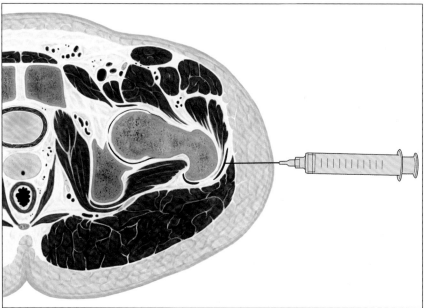

Figure 8.1 Trochanteric bursitis.

ISCHIOGLUTEAL BURSITIS (HAMSTRING TENDINOPATHY)

This condition is characterised by pain felt deeply in the buttock over the ischial tuberosity and aggravated by sitting, especially on hard surfaces. The medial area of this bony prominence is covered with fibro-fatty substance that contains the ischial bursa of the gluteus maximus muscle. The bursa lies over the ischial tuberosity and the sciatic nerve. Because of the deep-seated pain experienced, it is often confused with sciatic pain, making a difficult differential diagnosis. On examination, straight leg raising is usually normal, but there is tenderness felt deeply in the buttock on palpation, and it may be possible to detect a fluctuant swelling.

Prolonged sitting on hard surfaces or a bicycle saddle may precipitate the condition.

Injection technique (see Figure 8.2)

With the patient lying prone or on the side with the hip flexed and the affected side uppermost, inject 1 ml of steroid mixed with 1 ml lidocaine 1% plain in a 2 ml syringe into the point of maximal tenderness. It is necessary to use a larger, 1.5 inch (3.8 cm), needle to reach the bursa. When the injection has been sited correctly, the pain and tenderness will be abolished immediately, on account of the local anaesthetic; this confirms that the diagnosis was indeed the correct one.

Ischial tuberosity

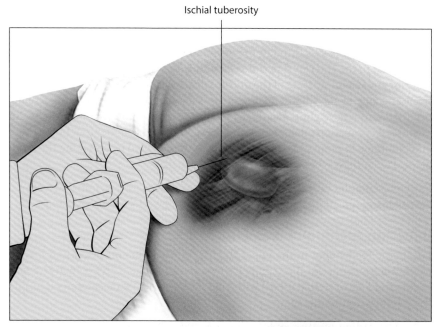

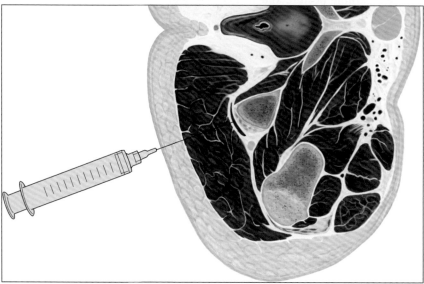

Figure 8.2 Ischiogluteal bursitis.

MERALGIA PARAESTHETICA

This entrapment syndrome is due to compression of the lateral cutaneous nerve of the thigh as it passes through the deep fascia about 3.9 inches (10 cm) below and medial to the anterior superior crest of the iliac spine. The nerve supplies the anterior and lateral surfaces of the mid-thigh. Typical paraesthesiae are felt in the front and side of the thigh, often after walking or prolonged standing. Usually occurring in overweight patients, the condition may be affected by a change in posture. Examination often reveals an area of numbness on the front of the thigh and bluntness to pinprick, and the diagnosis is confirmed by palpating the point of local tenderness where the nerve enters the thigh.

Early presentation of this syndrome may be mistaken for the initial stages of a herpes zoster infection; it may be wise to wait for 2 weeks before injecting.

Injection technique (see Figure 8.3)

Locate the tender spot in the upper thigh 3.9 inches (10 cm) below and medial to the anterior superior iliac spine. Using a 2 ml syringe with a 1 inch (2.5 cm) needle and 1 ml of steroid mixed with 1 ml lidocaine 1% plain, carefully infiltrate the solution around this spot.

Advice regarding posture and weight reduction is useful in preventing recurrences of the condition. Chronic cases occasionally require surgical referral for division of the lateral cutaneous nerve.

It may be appropriate to consider an ultrasound-guided injection for this condition if symptoms fail to improve after a non-guided injection.

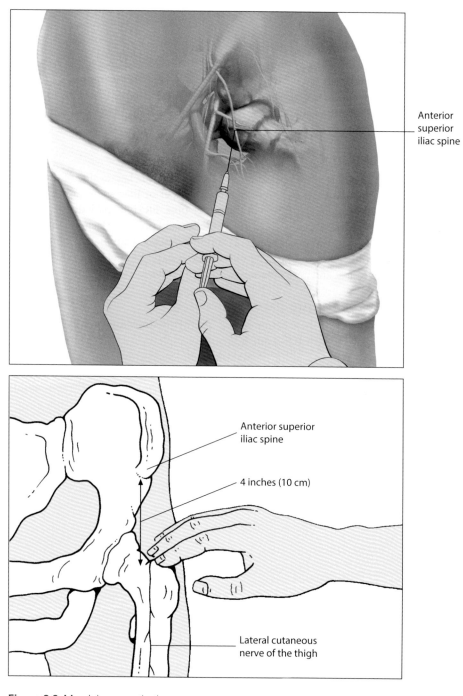

Figure 8.3 Meralgia paraesthetica.

ILIOTIBIAL BAND FRICTION SYNDROME

Presentation and diagnosis

This overuse injury is commonly seen in long distance runners, cyclists and skiers and, occasionally, in golfers and walkers. Males are more commonly affected. Pain occurs at the lateral side of the knee joint superior to the joint line and often radiates up the lateral side of the thigh. There is a point of maximal tenderness over the lateral femoral condyle.

Functional anatomy

The iliotibial band is a thickening of the fascia lata in the lateral side of the thigh. It is superficial and extends from the anterior superior iliac spine to the Gerdy's tubercle on the anterolateral side of the upper tibia. Flexion and extension of the knee joint causes the band to move in an anterior and posterior fashion, thus causing friction of the band over the lateral femoral condyle. Pain may be quite acute, which is an indication to inject steroid. Otherwise, physiotherapy in the form of deep massage, heat and anti-inflammatories are useful.

Injection technique (see Figure 8.4)

Inject 0.5–1 ml of hexacetonide or methylprednisolone acetate (Depo-Medrone®) mixed with 0.5–1 ml lidocaine 1% plain, using a 1 inch (2.5 cm) blue hub needle at the point of maximal tenderness, over the lateral side of the femoral condyle, after making a thumbnail imprint to identify the point of injection. Occasionally, a bursa is present posterior to the insertion, and it should also be injected.

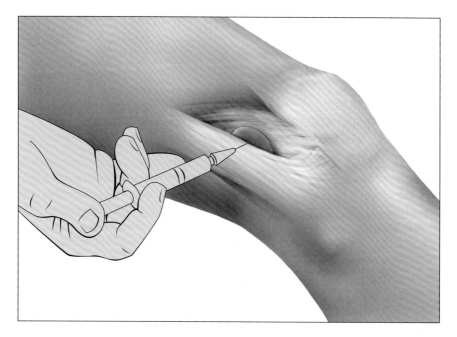

Figure 8.4 Iliotibial band syndrome.

PHYSIOTHERAPY: CONDITIONS AROUND THE HIP AND THIGH

Trochanteric bursitis

Physiotherapy treatment for GTPS aims at addressing the underlying abductor/ external rotator tendinosis. For acutely painful symptoms, steroid injection is extremely effective. Alternatives to injection include avoidance of painful activity, strapping, ice packs, analgesia, NSAIDs, soft tissue therapy and acupuncture.

However, to avoid recurrence, the ability of the tendon to transfer load needs to be improved in order to return to full activity without exacerbating pain. A progressive rehabilitation programme can be provided by a physiotherapist and is particularly important in recurrent or chronic cases. This programme may include exercises such as standing on one leg, stepping up and down from a stair or walking as simple ways of exercising the glutei. All should be carried out at a level that avoids exacerbating pain as the amount of exercise is steadily increased over several months, until the patient is back to full function. Compression of the tendons over the greater trochanter should also be avoided (e.g. prolonged sitting or sitting with crossed legs).

Ischiogluteal bursitis

Ischiogluteal bursitis is relatively uncommon and, as already stated, differentiating the diagnosis is challenging. The cause of the bursitis will help guide physiotherapy and other treatment.

Acute bursitis caused by the trauma of a fall on the buttock can be eased by cold therapy, analgesia and avoiding painful activity. These measures can also aid acute symptoms caused by repetitive overuse, which is typically increased running distance, pace or difficulty of terrain. Correction of a poor running pattern and addressing weakness and poor flexibility in the gluteal and hamstring muscles will help to reduce friction between the bursa and overlying structures.

Patients who have lost the 'padding' of the buttock due to significant weight loss or following complex hip surgery can suffer from bursitis as a result of direct pressure on the ischial tuberosity when sitting. The benefit of the injection can be enhanced by the patient sitting on soft cushions with pressure taken through the thighs rather than the tuberosity. Regular gluteal contractions (buttock clenching) and regular relief of the pressure by standing and walking can help prevent recurrence.

Meralgia paraesthetica

Physiotherapy is not usually required for this condition, which involves a purely sensory nerve. Prevention includes weight loss, avoiding sitting with the hip flexed beyond 90 degrees and avoiding tight clothing constricting the area.

Iliotibial band friction syndrome

In common with all overuse conditions, a long-term goal of treatment is to address the underlying cause and prevent recurrence. Comprehensive assessment of the lower limb and pelvis may be needed to identify these issues.

Correct footwear, good muscle strength and soft tissue flexibility can optimise the biomechanics of the lower limb and reduce the friction between the ilio-tibial band and underlying femoral condyle. Running shoes should be replaced regularly so that they provide support and good impact absorption. Athletes with poor foot posture, including a pronated or supinated foot, can benefit from orthotic assessment.

Gluteal strengthening exercises will improve the position of the femur during the heel strike and stance phase of gait and running. Weakness of these hip muscles causes increased adduction of the femur and has been associated with anterior knee pain including iliotibial band friction syndrome.

Soft tissue mobilisation of the iliotibial band and glutei by a physiotherapist or sport therapist can be reinforced by home treatment using a foam roller.

Evaluation of sporting activity can highlight specific issues to address. For example, cyclists may need to change the position of the saddle and cleat clips to improve the flexion/extension/rotation movement around the knee. Similar measures for runners include changing a running route to reduce prolonged downhill distances and banked surfaces.

REFERENCE

1 Rompe JD *et al* (2009) Home training, local corticosteroid injection, or radial shock wave therapy for greater trochanter pain syndrome. *Am J Sports Med.* **37** (10): 1981–1990.

CHAPTER 9

The knee joint

INTRODUCTION

Effusions of the knee joint are commonly seen in general practice, and both aspiration and steroid injection may be confidently undertaken.

There are many causes of effusion, such as trauma, strained collateral ligaments, cruciate and meniscus tears, haemarthrosis, rheumatoid disease, osteoarthritis, Reiter's syndrome, gout, pseudogout, psoriasis and, rarely, chondromalacia patellae.

Prepatellar and infrapatellar bursae ('clergyman's' and 'housemaid's' knees), occur because of recurrent pressure or trauma of kneeling and should not be confused with effusion of the knee joint. Prepatellar bursitis was more common in coal miners and carpet layers. These latter are prone to infection and must be distinguished from effusion of the knee joint. Osteochondritis dissecans, causing loose bodies in the knee joint, may lead to effusion and locking of the joint. A posterior Baker's cyst may rupture during violent flexion of the joint. This may occur in rheumatoid arthritis.

PRESENTATION AND DIAGNOSIS

An effusion is often detected on inspection and both knees should be inspected with the patient first standing and then lying on the couch.

Palpate the patella for the following signs:

- With an effusion, the hollows alongside the kneecap disappear, and a suprapatellar bulge may appear that is painful on palpation. The 'patella tap' may be less painful with smaller effusions, but the fluid can be stroked from one side of the patella to the other.
- Synovial thickening, which may be nodular, indicates synovitis.
- Bony prominences (osteophytes), which may occur in osteoarthritis.
- Note the temperature, by placing the backs of the fingers on the patella. In infection and crystal synovitis, there will be warmth, tenderness and redness of the overlying skin.
- Patellar 'grating' and crepitus, which occur in osteoarthritis.

Examine the full active and passive movements of the knee joint and note any quadriceps wasting.

FUNCTIONAL ANATOMY

The knee joint is a hinge joint and a major weight-bearing joint. The joint cavity is large and is essentially the patella-condylar space; it communicates with the suprapatellar and infrapatellar bursae.

ASPIRATION AND INJECTION THERAPY

There are three indications for aspiration of an effusion of the knee joint:

1 *Diagnostic*, in septic arthritis, haemarthrosis, traumatic effusion, rheumatoid arthritis, osteoarthritis, gout and pseudogout. Send the aspirate to the laboratory for analysis (Table 9.1).

2 *Therapeutic*, when a tense effusion causes pain and discomfort.

3 (a) *Steroid injection* for an acute flare-up, for example, of rheumatoid arthritis, osteoarthritis, psoriasis, Reiter's syndrome, synovitis and soft tissue lesions that occur in trauma; (b) *viscosupplementation* with hyaluronic acid preparation in osteoarthritis.

Trauma that may be quite minor, as occurs on the playing field, may often produce a large effusion into the knee joint, and as much as 60–70 ml of fluid may be aspirated. Should the effusion recur in the following 2 weeks, it is good practice to re-aspirate.

Due to advances in orthopaedic surgery, the management of rheumatoid arthritis and osteoarthritis affecting the knee and hip joints has changed considerably, mainly due to the success of total joint replacement. Osteoarthritis has become increasingly common in younger athletes (especially those who have required meniscus surgery), in whom joint replacement may not be appropriate because of their young age. Here, steroid injections may well tide them over until they reach an age when total joint replacement is more appropriate. Both these therapeutic regimes are suitable for a flare-up of an osteoarthritic knee joint that presents with pain, or a warm or hot painful joint that is not responding to NSAIDs. An acute exacerbation of seropositive or seronegative arthropathy due to rheumatoid or psoriatic arthropathy, for instance, will respond dramatically to an injection of triamcinolone acetonide, with remission often lasting for 6–12 months.

In recent years, there has been an increasing interest in viscosupplementation in the treatment of osteoarthritis of the knees.[1] This treatment has been largely used in Canada and Europe, and presents an alternative treatment for this condition.

Table 9.1 Analysis of synovial fluid

Diagnosis	Appearance	Viscosity	Special findings
Normal	Clear yellow	High	–
Traumatic	Straw to red	High	Blood may be ++
Osteoarthritis	Clear yellow	High	Cartilage fragments
Gout	Cloudy	Decreased	Monosodium urate crystals (needle-like)
Pseudogout	Cloudy	Decreased	Calcium pyrophosphate crystals (rhomboid)
Rheumatoid arthritis (RA)	Greenish, cloudy	Low	Latex RA haemagglutination titre or sheep cell agglutination test
Septic arthritis	Turbid to purulent	Low	Culture positive
TB (tuberculosis) arthritis	Cloudy	Low	Culture positive for acid-test bacillus

At the time of the fifth edition, this was a promising therapeutic option; but current NICE guidelines in the UK have shown that evidence is limited in supporting the use of this therapeutic option. It is not currently supported for clinical use.

Inject with steroids no more than once every 3 months. This is most effective for acute flare-ups of arthropathy, especially those that affect a single joint, as in psoriasis or rheumatoid arthritis exacerbations. Unlike steroids, a viscosupplementation course of three injections in 3 weeks may be repeated twice in 1 year.

TECHNIQUE OF ASPIRATION AND INJECTION (SEE FIGURE 9.1)

The patient lies on the couch with the knee slightly flexed; a pillow behind the knee is helpful. This allows relaxation of the quadriceps and patellar tendon. Carefully palpate the bony margin of the patella, which may be moved freely before the needle is inserted. Injection can be from either the lateral or the medial side of the patella and below the superior border of the patella.

Aspiration

- Prepare a 20 ml (or 50 ml) syringe and a sterile specimen container for diagnostic microscopy and culture. Use a 1.5 inch (3.8 cm) needle.
- Insert the needle horizontally and in a slightly downward (or posterior) direction into the joint, in the gap between the back of the patella and the femoral condyles. When the needle is behind the patella, it is in the joint space. Just before reaching that stage, it should be possible to slide the patella over the femur freely from side to side, ensuring relaxation of the quadriceps.
- If a steroid injection is to follow the aspiration, leave a small amount of synovial fluid in the knee joint. This will allow the steroid to diffuse around the joint cavity more easily.
- It is kinder, but not strictly necessary, to infiltrate 1 ml lidocaine 1% plain into the skin at the aspiration site.

Injection

- Use 1 ml of steroid (20 mg triamcinolone acetonide, 40 mg methylprednisolone or 20 mg hydrocortisone acetate) in a 2 ml syringe. Use a 1.5 inch (3.8 cm) needle.
- Follow the same needle insertion procedure as for aspiration, earlier.
- Inject steroid into the knee no more than once every 3 months.

After aspiration or injection, the knee joint should be rested for 24 hours, supported by a firm Tubigrip or elastic crêpe bandage.

The short-term benefit of intra-articular steroids in the treatment of osteoarthritis of the knee joint is well established and few side effects have been reported. Longer-term beneficial effects have not been confirmed.

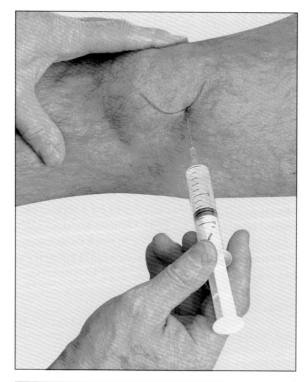

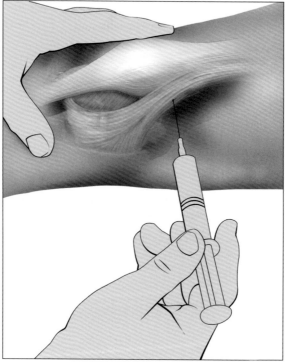

Figure 9.1 The knee joint.

PHYSIOTHERAPY: THE KNEE

Intra-articular steroid or hyaluronic acid injection is most commonly used to treat symptomatic osteoarthritis and is ideally placed within a package of care aimed at long-term management of this condition. Guidance published by the National Institute for Health and Care Excellence[2] recommends information on self-management, including weight loss for people who are overweight or obese, and use of supportive, shock-absorbing footwear and walking aids. Exercise is recommended for all patients. General and aerobic fitness can be improved without overloading the joint and exacerbating pain by exercise in water, cycling or gym-based circuits. Specific exercise to improve muscle strength, joint flexibility and proprioception can be prescribed by a physiotherapist.

Simple analgesia, taken either prior to activity or on a regular basis, can be supplemented by topical NSAIDS or capsaicin. The use of oral NSAIDs remains controversial, but short-term use can assist in limiting an acute exacerbation. A knee effusion caused by trauma, degenerative change or inflammatory arthritis can be assisted by use of cold packs.

REFERENCES

1   Balaz EA and Denliger JL (1993) Viscosupplementation: a new concept in the treatment of os teoarthritis. *J Rheumatol.* **20** (39): 3–9.

2   National Institute for Health and Care Excellence: Clinical Guidelines [Internet]. London, UK: National Institute for Health and Care Excellence (UK); 2014. Available from: https://www.nice.org.uk/guidance/cg177 [accessed 8/10/18].

FURTHER READING

Bagga H *et al* (2006) Long-term effects of intra-articular hyaluronan on synovial fluid in osteoarthritis of the knee. *J Rheumatol.* **33**: 946–950.

Bellamy N *et al* (2006) Intra-articular corticosteroid for treatment of osteoarthritis of the knee. *Cochrane Database Syst Rev.* **2**: CD005328.

Dickson DJ and Hosie G (1998) *Poster at BSR Conference*, Brighton, UK.

Gossec L and Dougados M (2006) Do intra-articular therapies work and who will benefit most? *Best Pract Res Clin Rheumatol.* **20**: 131–144.

Petrella RJ and Petrella M (2006) A prospective, randomized, double-blind, placebo controlled study to evaluate the efficacy of intra-articular hyaluronic acid for osteoarthritis of the knee. *J Rheumatol.* **33**: 951–956.

CHAPTER 10

The ankle and foot

INTRODUCTION

Disorders of the foot and ankle are increasingly common in general practice, owing to the popularity of sports and physical training, in particular jogging. Ankle sprains, the most common injury in general practice, have an estimated episode rate of 28 per 2500 patients per year.

FUNCTIONAL ANATOMY

The ankle joint is a simple hinge joint, allowing only simple plantar and dorsiflexion. The joint is supported by a fibrous capsule, a lateral (calcaneofibular) and a medial (deltoid) ligament, and anterior and posterior ligaments. The tibialis anterior muscle, assisted by the extensor digitorum longus and extensor hallucis longus, account for dorsiflexion. Plantar flexion is brought about by the gastrocnemius and soleus, assisted by the plantaris, tibialis posterior, flexor hallucis longus and flexor digitorum longus muscles. The other main movements of the foot are eversion and inversion, which take place at the talocalcaneal, talonavicular and calcaneocuboid joints. The latter two together form the mid-tarsal joint. The forefoot, involving the heads of the metatarsals, is the site of many painful conditions, known collectively as metatarsalgia.

PRESENTATION OF SOME COMMON PROBLEMS

- *Lateral ligament sprains.* Sprains as a result of inversion injury cause a complete or partial tear of the lateral ligament. Pain and swelling may be considerable, leading to difficulty in accurate assessment of the damage.

- *Achilles tendon.* Rupture is characterised by sudden and severe pain in the calf (as if being suddenly kicked from behind), in the absence of any obvious injury. The tear may be palpated and the patient is unable to stand on the toes of the affected foot. Immediate referral for suture or immobilisation is indicated. Achilles tendinosis is caused by inflammation of the tendon at the insertion into the calcaneum or along the length of the tendon, or in the bursa separating the tendon from the calcaneum. Crepitus may be felt, as in any other form of tenosynovitis. The popularity of jogging has increased the incidence of these problems. It should be noted that tendon inflammation and rupture are a recognised complication, occurring rarely, during therapy with some quinolone antibiotics (e.g. ciprofloxacin). The reason for this is not understood, but the author can confirm from personal experience the rupture of two posterior tibial tendons and one Achilles tendon following medication with ciprofloxacin. In any patient considered to be prone to tendinosis problems or similar tenosynovitis problems, avoidance of such antibiotic prescription must be advised.[1]

- *Plantar fasciitis.* This painful heel condition is characterised by an acutely tender spot in the middle of the heel pad on standing or walking. There is often a calcaneal spur demonstrated on a radiograph of the heel. This condition may occur in the seronegative arthropathies and should be suspected if the radiograph also demonstrates erosions or a fluffy or irregular calcaneal spur.

In the past, radiographs were obtained to identify the presence of a heel spur, but it is well established that the presence or absence of a heel spur bears little relationship to the diagnosis of plantar fasciitis.

In refractory cases, ultrasound is helpful in providing objective confirmation based on the thickness of the plantar fascia; it may be useful to undertake a guided injection into the paratenon and avoid the risk of rupture due to repeated injections into the substance of the plantar fascia[2-5].

- *Tarsal tunnel syndrome.* This is an uncommon condition of posterior tibial nerve entrapment as it passes under the flexor retinaculum, and is analogous to the carpal tunnel syndrome of the wrist. The patient will complain of paroxysmal paraesthesia, numbness and pain along the medial border of the foot, the great toe and the distal part of the sole.

- *The ankle and mid-tarsal joint.* The ankle and the mid-tarsal joint may be affected by rheumatoid arthritis, with the subtalar joint being more commonly affected. Seronegative arthropathies, such as Reiter's syndrome, psoriasis and ankylosing spondylitis, may affect the small mid-tarsal joints of the foot.

- *The forefoot.* This is involved in the many causes of metatarsalgia, especially pes cavus, March fracture, hallux rigidus and Morton's neurofibroma. Also, in the elderly, the fatty pad of the sole may degenerate, causing the patient to complain that it is like 'walking on marbles'. Rheumatoid arthritis and gout may affect the forefoot, the latter condition most commonly affecting the first metatarsal joint of the great toe. Toe deformities such as hallux rigidus, hammer toes, claw toes and bunions all cause metatarsalgia.

INJECTION TECHNIQUE (SEE FIGURE 10.1)

Ankle sprains

These are best treated with the standard management of 'RICE': rest, ice, compression and elevation. This will help to provide pain relief and reduce inflammation and swelling. Physiotherapy referral is appropriate.

Injections in this setting are not performed routinely, as steroid may cause further damage to injured tendons.

Refractory symptoms indicate specialist review, as significant ligamentous or chondral injury may be associated with premature osteoarthritis if overlooked.

Achilles tendon

Although steroid injections have been described for treating Achilles tendinopathy with extreme caution, general practitioners (GPs) are advised to refrain from this treatment. The relief is so often only temporary and the possibility of Achilles tendon rupture so likely that the advice is to refer these problems for specialist care. Unfortunately, the incidence of litigation is high, and GPs are advised to diagnose Achilles tendon problems with care, never to inject steroid into the substance of a tendon and preferably to seek the advice of a specialist in these cases.

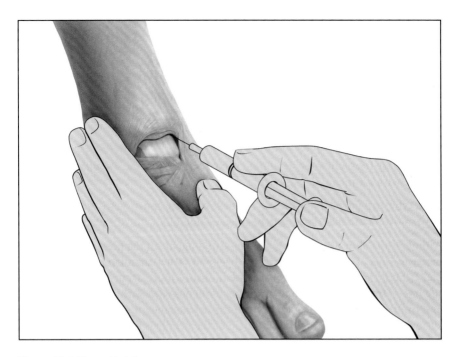

Figure 10.1 The ankle joint.

PLANTAR FASCIITIS: THE PAINFUL HEEL

The painful heel is an acutely tender spot in the middle of the heel pad, which can be accurately palpated by firm pressure. The pain is due to plantar fasciitis, which is a strain of the long plantar ligament at its insertion into the calcaneum. The condition may occur alone or in other forms of arthritis, such as Reiter's disease and ankylosing spondylitis.

Injection technique (see Figure 10.2)

Use 1 ml of triamcinolone acetonide mixed with lidocaine 1% plain in a 2 ml syringe with a 1 inch (2.5 cm) needle.

Allow the patient to lie prone on the examination couch with the heel facing uppermost. First swab the area to be injected liberally with 70% alcohol.

Although the skin of the heel is thicker and tougher on the plantar surface, it is better to inject from the centre of the heel pad rather than from the side of the pad (where the skin is thinner). This will ensure more accurate localisation of the injection. Infiltrate the skin and subcutaneous area with lidocaine 1% plain and infiltrate lidocaine deeply down to the calcaneal spur, and then change the syringe leaving the needle *in situ*; the tip of the needle is accurately placed at the point of maximum tenderness, often touching the periosteum, before 0.5–1 ml of steroid mixed with 1 ml 1% lidocaine solution is injected. The whole lesion should preferably be infiltrated by moving the needle point to each tender spot to cover the whole lesion – as described for tennis elbow.

Since this is a painful injection, it is best to mix the steroid solution with lidocaine and infiltrate the skin as much as possible while, at the same time, advancing the needle towards the most tender spot. As the duration of action of lidocaine is only between 2 and 4 hours, bupivacaine plain 0.25% or 0.5% may be used instead of the lidocaine in recurrent cases. As the duration of action of bupivacaine may last for up to 16 hours, it is often kinder for the patient as it provides an anaesthetic effect until the anti-inflammatory effect of the steroid takes over.

Simple analgesia, avoiding walking on the affected heel for a couple of days and, perhaps, wearing a sponge rubber heel pad for a few days is sound post-injection advice.

TARSAL TUNNEL SYNDROME

This condition may also be treated with steroid injection, as for carpal tunnel syndrome in the wrist. The needle is inserted posterior to the flexor retinaculum behind the medial malleolus, between that and the calcaneus of the ankle joint.

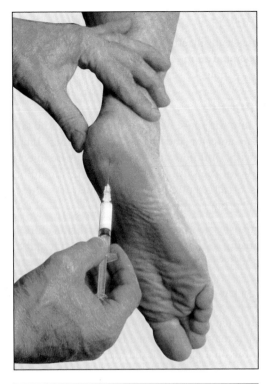

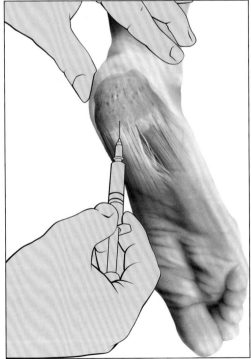

Figure 10.2 Plantar fasciitis.

THE ANKLE JOINT

The anterior approach to injection and aspiration is the simplest and the only approach that GPs should adopt. Flare-ups of arthropathies respond well to injection of this joint. Care must be scrupulously exercised to avoid infection.

Injection technique

Insert the needle into the space between the tibia and the talus anteriorly, and between the tibialis anterior and the extensor hallucis longus tendons; 1 ml of steroid mixed with 1 ml lidocaine 1% plain may be injected using a 1 inch (2.5 cm) needle. As for the knee joint, any aspirate should be sent for microscopy and analysis. Strict aseptic precautions must be adhered to as the ankle joint is particularly prone to infection.

In addition to corticosteroid injection for osteoarthritis of the ankle joint, viscosupplementation, using sodium hyaluronate, has been found to be effective. The latter will provide sustained relief of pain and improve ankle function.[6]

TIBIALIS POSTERIOR TENDINOSIS

This strain is due to a tenosynovitis of the tendon sheath. Usually a sports injury (e.g. in footballers), it may also be caused by a simple strain such as working on a ladder and reaching on a plantar flexed foot. It may also occur in rheumatoid arthritis. The pain is reproduced by inversion of the plantar flexed foot. Crepitus may be palpable along the line of the tendon sheath, especially directly posterior and inferior to the medial malleolus.

Functional anatomy

This muscle arises from the lateral part of the posterior surface of the tibia, the interosseous membrane and the adjoining part of the fibula. It is thus the deepest muscle in the calf. The tendon then becomes more superficial and grooves the posterior surface of the lower end of the tibia and lies behind and directly below the medial malleolus. It then passes forward under the flexor retinaculum into the sole of the foot. It is inserted into the tuberosity of the navicular bone and gives off slips, which pass to the calcaneum, the cuboid, the three cuneiform bones and the bases of the second, third and fourth metatarsals.

A strain of this tendon may produce pain in the ankle and foot anywhere along the course of the tendon or in any of its attachments in the foot.

Injection technique (see Figure 10.3)

Use a small needle, 1.6 cm, with a 2 ml syringe containing 0.5–1.0 ml of triamcinolone acetonide mixed with 1 ml lidocaine 1% plain. Place the fingers of the left hand on the tendon sheath immediately behind the medial malleolus to steady the tendon, and inject the needle in line with the tendon below the medial malleolus and in a proximal direction. As in the earlier descriptions of other forms of tenosynovitis injection, it is preferable to place the needle deeply into the substance of the tendon, when the doctor will immediately notice resistance

Tibialis posterior
tendon and sheath

Medial malleolus

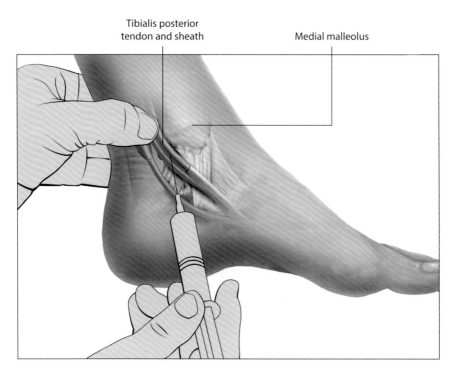

Figure 10.3 Tibialis posterior tendinosis.

to the injection. Then, while maintaining pressure on the syringe plunger as if to inject, gradually withdraw the needle and syringe until the moment that no resistance to injection is felt; the needle is now in the tendon sheath space. Then, inject up to 2 ml of the mixture.

It is helpful for the patient to rest the foot and ankle for a few days after the injection and to wear an elastic ankle support for up to 6 weeks. The only physiotherapy adjunct to treatment that is helpful is deep friction twice weekly for 3 or 4 weeks.

PHYSIOTHERAPY: THE ANKLE AND FOOT

Ankle sprains

The pain and swelling of an acute lateral ligament injury are effectively treated with the standard management of 'POLICE': Protection, Optimal Loading, Ice, Compression and Elevation. The term 'optimal loading' refers to the use of early pain-free movement, which incrementally increases with recovery to include the addition of load and stress through the healing structures. Physiotherapy referral is appropriate to facilitate this.

Plantar fasciitis

Predisposing factors to plantar fasciitis include a high body mass index (BMI), poor or worn footwear, reduced or increased medial foot arch, and excessive standing or impact activity. Addressing these issues with a weight loss programme, use of generic or custom-made orthotics and shock-absorbing insoles can reduce the risk of recurrence.

The plantar fascia is continuous with that of the Achilles tendon and both can be mobilised by calf stretches performed with the big toe in a dorsiflexed position. The supporting structure provided by the bony foot arches can be enhanced by strengthening the small intrinsic foot muscles.

Where the fasciitis is causing sleep disturbance, use of a splint can help to maintain the foot in a more comfortable position of dorsiflexion.

Chronic or recurrent cases may require additional advice from a podiatrist or physiotherapist.

Tarsal tunnel

Conservative treatment aims to resolve inflammation and, therefore, prevent long-term compromise of the posterior tibial nerve. In addition to injection, advice on avoidance of provocative activities, cold therapy, NSAIDs, foot strapping, and use of supportive footwear will facilitate prompt resolution.

Identifying the underlying causes is important in a more established condition. Foot deformity, secondary to arthritis or extreme flat foot, can lead to neural compression. Improving foot posture with well-fitting shoes or orthotics can help improve symptoms.

Ankle arthritis

The principles underlying conservative management of ankle arthritis are identical to those at the knee (*see* Chapter 9).

Tibialis posterior tendinosis

The clinical presentation of a patient with tibialis posterior tendinosis can range from acute tenosynovitis in a recreational athlete to a chronic degenerative tear associated with a significant flat foot deformity.

Treatment in acute tendinosis includes avoidance of painful activity (with short-term use of crutches, if necessary), strapping, cold therapy and gradual introduction of exercises to restore normal movement, strength and balance.

In recurrent or chronic conditions, a podiatrist or physiotherapist will also address predisposing factors. Shoes and/or orthotics to support the medial arch of the foot will improve foot posture on weight bearing. In all cases of tendinopathy, rehabilitation to improve the ability of the tendon to transfer load is vital. Strengthening, stretching and balance exercise for the ankle will improve the function of the tibialis posterior in controlling deceleration of pronation and dorsiflexion when walking or running. Non-weight-bearing exercise is gradually progressed to functional weight-bearing work and, finally to multidirectional speed and ballistic activity, provided symptoms are not being exacerbated.

REFERENCES

1 Association of British Pharmaceutical Industry (1999) *ABPI Compendium of Data Sheets and Summaries of Product Characteristics 1999–2000 with the Code of Practice for the Pharmaceutical Industry*. Datapharm Publication, London, UK, p. 167.

2 Johal KS and Milner SA (2012) Plantar fasciitis and the calcaneal spur: fact or fiction? *Foot Ankle Surgery*. **18**: 39–41.

3 Sellman JR (1994) Plantar fascia rupture associated with corticosteroid injection. *Foot Ankle Int*. **15**: 376–381.

4 McMillan AM *et al* (2009) Diagnostic imaging for chronic plantar heel pain: a systematic review and meta-analysis. *J Foot Ankle Res*. **2**: 32.

5 Gibbon WW and Long G (1999) Ultrasound of the plantar aponeurosis (fascia). *Skeletal Radiol*. **28** (1): 21.

6 Salk R *et al* (2005) Viscosupplementation (hyaluronans) in the treatment of ankle osteoarthritis. *Clin Podiatr Med Surg N Am*. **22**: 585–597.

CHAPTER 11

Musculoskeletal imaging and therapeutic options in soft tissue disorders

INTRODUCTION

The content of this manual has so far concentrated on the clinical diagnosis and management of soft tissue and joint disorders. Soft tissue complaints are extremely common in general practice consultations, and shoulder pain alone is a common complaint, with a reported prevalence of 6.9%–34% in the general population and 21% in those over 70 years of age. It accounts for 1.2% of all general practice encounters. Uncertainty remains regarding the relative merits and efficacy for all available therapies, with little in the way of evidence-based practice available.

Training has traditionally focused on history taking, examination and clinical diagnosis, and this remains the mainstay of patient management in soft tissue disorders. Over the past decade, the imaging of soft tissue and joint disorders has progressed dramatically with the advent of magnetic resonance imaging (MRI) and, more latterly, ultrasound. This has led to a significant change in the understanding of musculoskeletal disorders and the underlying biomechanical derangement. This added information can therefore be translated into clinically-oriented problem solving, allowing confident diagnosis and effective management strategies, which will benefit patients in terms of treatment, prevention and effective management beyond the primary care setting. Imaging allows thinking to progress and allows exploration of the 'cause of the cause' (i.e. the underlying biomechanical disorder). Given that soft tissue and joint disorders account for a significant proportion of consultations in general practice and hospital outpatient clinics, this part of training is sadly neglected at undergraduate and postgraduate levels.

PATHOPHYSIOLOGY

An understanding of the pathophysiology and biomechanics of tendon disorders is fundamental to diagnosis and treatment. Imaging has led to greater knowledge and understanding of these disorders, allowing a more critical approach to their diagnosis and treatment. It should be stressed, however, that despite the power of complex imaging to demonstrate subtle tendon abnormalities, the appropriate imaging strategy and the significance of findings may not always be clear.

The terminology for tendon disorders has been confused in the past.

- *Tendinopathy* is a clinical description referring to both acute and chronic conditions.
- *Tendinosis* is a misnomer, as inflammatory cells are rarely seen histologically. The term refers to a non-inflammatory state with histological evidence of collagen disorganisation and necrosis.

Tendons without a synovial sheath (i.e. Achilles and plantar fascia) are surrounded by loose areolar tissue lined with synovial cells. This covering is called the paratenon; hence, when inflamed, it is called *paratenonitis*. Where a double synovial sheath is present (i.e. the tendons of the hands and feet) inflammation is referred to as *synovitis* (*see* Figure 11.1).

The aetiology of tendinosis is multifactorial and commonly related to repeated episodes of microtrauma, with breakdown of collagen cross-linking. If repair is incomplete, it may progress to further injury and tendon failure. This theory is supported by imaging the Achilles tendon of asymptomatic athletes where,

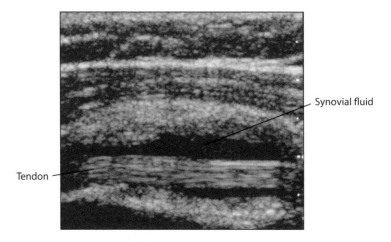

Synovial fluid

Tendon

Figure 11.1 Ultrasound scan showing tenosynovitis.

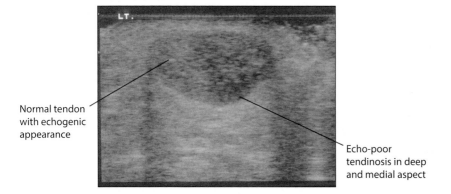

Normal tendon with echogenic appearance

Echo-poor tendinosis in deep and medial aspect

Figure 11.2 Transverse ultrasound scan of the Achilles tendon.

before rupture, there was a history of contralateral rupture. Features in keeping with tendinosis were found in 90%–95% of asymptomatic contralateral tendons. This suggests that tendon abnormalities exist that predispose to failure, thereby influencing the clinical management required to prevent further damage.

Steroid injections have been implicated as a risk factor in tendon rupture, but it is not possible to distinguish between tendons that have been injected and those that have not, either radiologically or pathologically. Therefore, while cortisone in and of itself may not pose a risk, its anti-inflammatory effect and role as a pain reliever may lead to the overloading of degenerate tendons. It is, however, considered unwise to inject directly into a tendon as the pressure effect may lead to hypoxia and degeneration.

The underlying biomechanical disorder can be deduced from the imaging findings in abnormal tendons – the Achilles tendon is a good example of where the distribution of abnormality within the tendon depends on the underlying problem (i.e. deep and medial with hyperpronation [*see* Figure 11.2] and superficial with high heel tabs). This information can be useful when prescribing corrective and preventive measures (i.e. treating the cause of the cause).

WHEN TO IMAGE

Injection techniques have been described in the previous chapters and the aim of this section is to add a further dimension to clinical practice. Not all practitioners will have confidence in making a precise diagnosis, addressing the underlying biomechanical disorder and treating it by way of advice or injection. In many instances, presentation may be 'atypical' and patients often request confirmation and traditional radiographic evidence. The use of plain film radiography in soft tissue diagnosis is limited because of the levels of radiation (levels that current European guidelines are trying to reduce). The imaging method of choice for soft tissue diagnosis is therefore either MRI or ultrasound, the latter of which carries no radiation burden. Advances in diagnostic ultrasound and its role in the resolution of soft tissue disorders means that it is now considered at least equal to or superior to MRI. It is also quicker to perform and less expensive.

As the popularity of sport and increased patient awareness of diagnostic and treatment options has led to increased demands on clinical practitioners, the option to image, with the added benefit of image-guided therapy, is now widely available to practitioners. While the majority of soft tissue disorders are either self-limiting or respond to conservative measures, including steroid injection, there are many instances where the diagnosis is unclear or the resolution of symptoms incomplete. Imaging strategies, therefore, offer an option for guidance without the need for traditional referral to orthopaedic clinics, whose main role is to identify surgical options.

IMAGING MODALITIES

Radiography

Plain film radiographs have an important role in demonstrating bone disorders of the shoulder (i.e. end-stage cuff arthropathy [see Figure 11.3] or showing erosive arthropathy [see Figure 11.4]), but have only a minor role in imaging soft tissue and tendon abnormalities. A good example is the 'heel spur' (see Figure 11.5). Radiography request is no longer considered justifiable in this case, as the presence or absence of a spur bears little relationship to associated plantar fasciitis, which is directly responsible for the pain. The spur is probably secondary to the underlying biomechanical disorder.

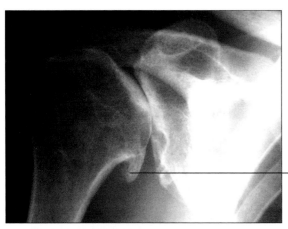

Figure 11.3 AP radiograph of the right shoulder demonstrating degenerative change secondary to rotator cuff failure ('cuff arthropathy').

Large inferior
humeral head
osteophyte

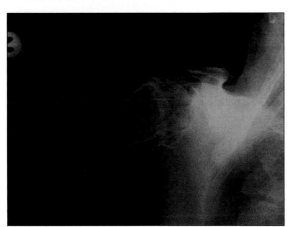

Figure 11.4 AP radiograph of the right shoulder showing erosions and destruction of the joint due to rheumatoid arthritis.

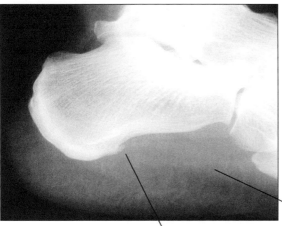

Figure 11.5 Lateral radiograph of the calcaneum showing a 'heel spur': this is often incidental but is also associated with seronegative arthropathy and Reiter's syndrome.

Plantar fascia

Inferior spur

Magnetic resonance imaging

MRI is widely used to image tendon and soft tissue pathology because the procedure avoids ionising radiation. While there is little doubt that MRI is a powerful tool, it is expensive, time consuming and not readily available. Requests for MRI are often best discussed with a musculoskeletal radiologist prior to referral, so that the appropriateness of the study and the best way of imaging the clinical problem can be achieved. Although well established for procedures such as rotator cuff imaging (*see* Figure 11.6), MRI has been superseded, to a degree, by modern ultrasound techniques.

Ultrasound

Advances in probe technology over the past 15 years have revolutionised the applications of ultrasound to the imaging of smaller structures in the near field, with spatial and contrast resolution now both at least as good as, or even better than, MRI. While most radiology departments are well equipped with ultrasound equipment, the equipment for musculoskeletal imaging has to be of the highest available standard with suitable high-frequency linear array probes. The equipment is also highly dependent on operator skill.

Advantages include the ability to image in real time, hence visualising abnormalities during painful movements. A good example is shoulder impingement, which has traditionally been a clinical diagnosis but can now be confirmed with dynamic scanning.

Ultrasound offers the opportunity for image-guided intervention (*see* Figure 11.7) and is used for biopsy, aspiration of fluid from synovial swellings or joints and direct placement of steroid and local anaesthetic into tendon sheaths and bursae where there is imaging evidence of abnormality.

Relative merits for different imaging modalities

Table 11.1 summarises the relative merits of the different imaging modalities.

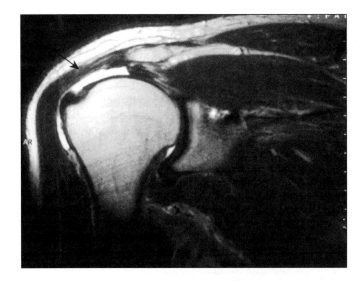

Figure 11.6 Coronal T2 MRI of the right shoulder demonstrating a full-thickness tear of the supraspinatus (arrow).

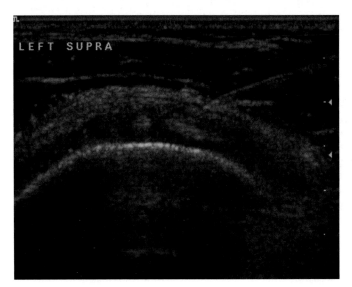

Figure 11.7 Ultrasound-guided injection of the subdeltoid bursa: note how thin the bursa is.

Table 11.1 Relative merits of different imaging modalities

	MRI	Ultrasound	Radiography
Bone	++	+	+++
Soft tissues	+++	++++	+
Guided injection	+	+++	+
Dynamic examination	+	++++	+
Cost	++++	+	+
Length of examination	++++	+	+

IMAGING OF JOINTS

General principles

Having decided to refer for imaging, it is helpful to provide the radiologist with a full clinical history and examination – he can then advise on the appropriate imaging modality and provide a report, which has maximum benefit to the general practitioner or clinician in assessing further management. It is often helpful for the practitioner to see an ultrasound scan performed so that he/she can understand the technique and appreciate its strengths and weaknesses.

It also provides an opportunity for revision of applied anatomy and pathophysiology of soft tissue disorders.

Before describing some practical examples, it should be stressed that all tendons have similar appearances on ultrasound examination, and general principles relating to abnormal appearances are similar at many sites. Ultrasound images presented in this chapter represent a 'snapshot' in time and are merely a record of a dynamic and interactive procedure.

The shoulder

The aetiology of rotator cuff tears is still debated, but it is primarily linked to advancing age. Other factors include impingement, deficiencies in collagen, relative avascularity and previous trauma. Shoulder pain is very common in clinical practice and patients present with a painful arc, radiation and, classically, night pain. There may be a history of trauma, which is often trivial in the elderly, and, typically, there is little response to physiotherapy, rest or injection if there is a rotator cuff tear.

The underlying disorder may be impingement associated with micro-instability in the younger age group or, more likely, a rotator cuff tear with increasing age, which almost always affects the supraspinatus. Subacromial bursitis is relatively rare, unless there is an underlying seropositive arthropathy with synovial proliferation. The presence of fluid on aspiration of the bursa should point to the presence of an underlying cuff tear. The intact cuff acts as a seal between the glenohumeral joint and the subdeltoid bursa and will, therefore, only distend in the presence of underlying cuff failure.

Time, rest and anti-inflammatories are the first-line treatments; only then, should injections of local anaesthetic and steroid be considered.

The use of ultrasound in diagnosing impingement and rotator cuff tears is well established and is probably superior to MRI, as it has the added advantage of dynamic testing and facilitates guided injections.

Lack of response to a single injection may signify an underlying tear, an incorrectly placed injection or a diagnosis that will not respond to subacromial injection. Ultrasound can be very useful in establishing the diagnosis in these cases and allows appropriate further management to be considered. With regard to rotator cuff tears, ultrasound will confirm impingement, distinguish partial from full-thickness tears and measure the size of full-thickness tears. This will have a direct impact on surgical planning. The term 'frozen shoulder' has been loosely applied in the past, and this disorder is quite unusual in clinical practice. The history of pain is important, as it tends to limit all movement, but pain typically presents on initiation of external rotation. Imaging is usually normal, and the underlying problem relates to adhesive capsulitis, particularly involving the rotator interval between the biceps and the leading edge of the supraspinatus. Treatment options include distension arthrography to break down capsular adhesions, or manipulation under anaesthesia. Interestingly, the abnormal tissue within the rotator interval is very similar, histologically, to Dupuytren's contracture (*see* Figures 11.8–11.15).

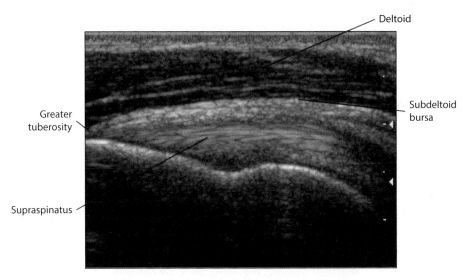

Figure 11.8 Longitudinal ultrasound scan demonstrating the normal supraspinatus.

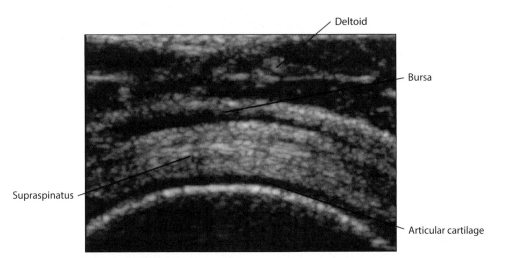

Figure 11.9 Transverse ultrasound scan demonstrating the normal supraspinatus.

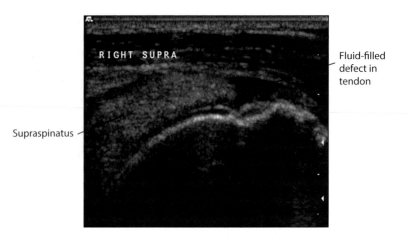

Fluid-filled
defect in
tendon

Supraspinatus

Figure 11.10 Ultrasound scan showing a full-thickness tear of the supraspinatus.

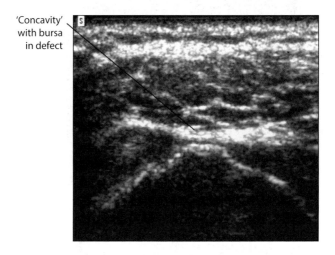

'Concavity'
with bursa
in defect

Figure 11.11 Full-thickness tear of the supraspinatus.

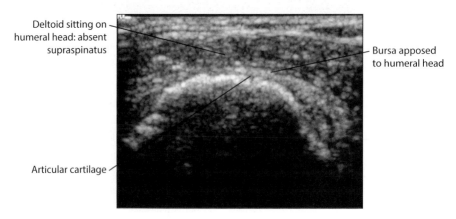

Deltoid sitting on
humeral head: absent
supraspinatus

Bursa apposed
to humeral head

Articular cartilage

Figure 11.12 Massive rotator cuff tear.

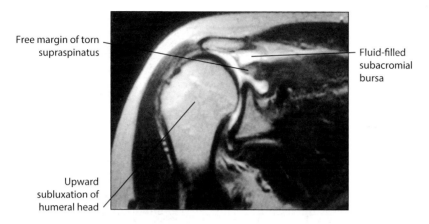

Free margin of torn supraspinatus

Fluid-filled subacromial bursa

Upward subluxation of humeral head

Figure 11.13 Coronal T2 MRI showing a complete tear of the supraspinatus.

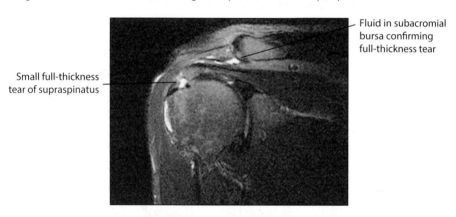

Fluid in subacromial bursa confirming full-thickness tear

Small full-thickness tear of supraspinatus

Figure 11.14 MRI arthrogram showing a supraspinatus tear.

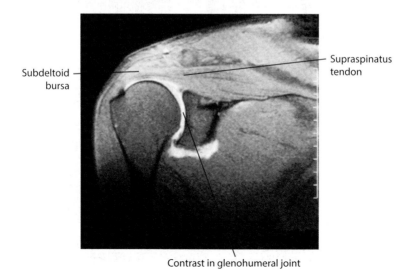

Subdeltoid bursa

Supraspinatus tendon

Contrast in glenohumeral joint

Figure 11.15 Coronal MRI with intra-articular contrast demonstrating an intact supraspinatus.

As the shoulder is clinically challenging, imaging has the following benefits:

- It excludes osteoarthritis.
- It excludes inflammatory arthritis.
- It allows diagnosis of rotator cuff tears.
- It can measure the size of the tear.
- It excludes biceps dislocation.
- It excludes calcific tendinosis.
- It allows the diagnosis of occult fractures.

Achilles tendon

The Achilles tendon is the most frequently injured ankle tendon, with injuries commonly occurring in a zone of relative avascularity 2–6 cm from the calcaneal insertion. Clinical diagnosis of complete rupture is usually straightforward.

Histologically, degenerative changes are present in a high percentage of spontaneous ruptures.

Ultrasound is a reliable method for imaging the abnormal Achilles tendon, and with complete rupture, the diagnosis can be confirmed and the distraction gap measured, which is useful in the operative assessment (*see* Figure 11.16). Plantaris tendon can be identified, which, if present, can lead to false-negative clinical tests for complete rupture. Following conservative or surgical management, ultrasound is useful for following the healing process and detecting complications.

Chronic Achilles pathology is more of a clinical challenge, and ultrasound will distinguish tendinosis, partial tear and chronic rupture (*see* Figure 11.17). Metabolic disease is quite common and intratendinous gouty tophi may be identified as a cause of pain, therefore allowing appropriate management.

The distribution of abnormality within the tendon allows a biomechanical understanding. Superficial changes associated with a pre-Achilles bursa 'pump–bump' suggest friction between the calcaneus and high heel tabs, as in Haglund's disease.

Deep and medial tendinosis suggests hyperpronation and deep and superficial tendinosis suggests muscle imbalance with abnormal loading.

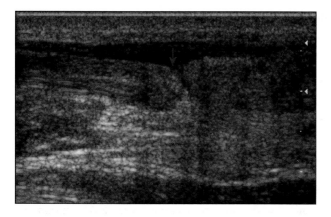

Figure 11.16 Ultrasound scan showing a complete tear of the Achilles tendon (arrow).

Fusiform
thickening in
tendinitis

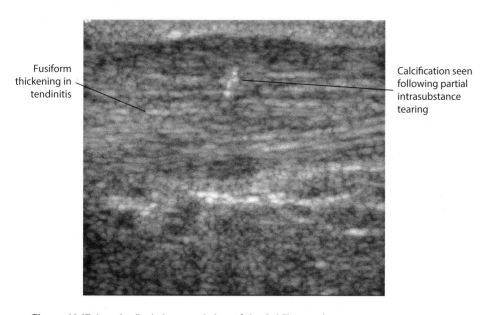

Calcification seen
following partial
intrasubstance
tearing

Figure 11.17 Longitudinal ultrasound view of the Achilles tendon.

The ankle

The static stabilisers (medial and lateral ligaments) are poorly visible on ultrasound. Injuries are usually managed without the need to image, unless symptoms persist. The dynamic stabilisers (peroneal and medial complex) are more clearly visible. The tibialis posterior is prone to significant degeneration, and complete ruptures are frequently overlooked.

The sequela of untreated rupture includes pes planus, hindfoot valgus, forefoot abduction and mid-tarsal degeneration. Tears usually occur around the medial malleolus or at the navicular insertion and cause medial ankle pain, pes planus and an inability to perform a single heel raise. Diagnosis is clearly important in order to prevent long-term disability (*see* Figures 11.18 and 11.19).

Partial tears may be traumatic or secondary to tibial osteophyte formation. Not uncommonly, there is a contralateral pes planus deformity, leading to overload on the affected side. Both ultrasound and MRI are useful tools in depicting tibialis tendinopathy and tears, thereby allowing early referral before rupture occurs.

Ultrasound-guided injection can be effective in treating symptoms of tibialis posterior tendinosis, allowing accurate steroid placement into the tendon sheath and avoiding tendon injection where early tenosynovitis is clinically undetectable.

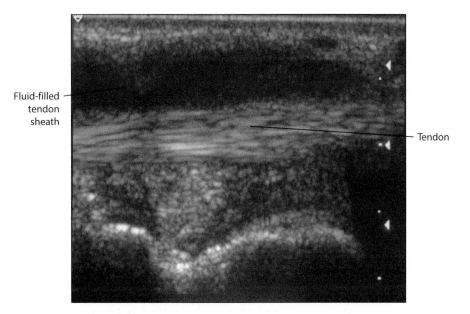

Fluid-filled tendon sheath

Tendon

Figure 11.18 Ultrasound scan demonstrating tibialis posterior tenosynovitis.

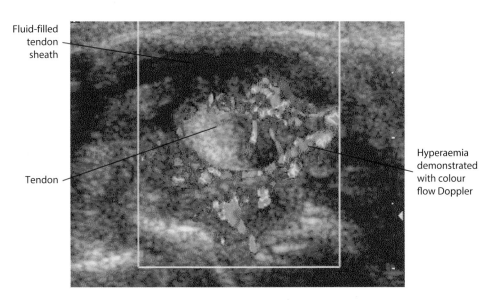

Fluid-filled tendon sheath

Tendon

Hyperaemia demonstrated with colour flow Doppler

Figure 11.19 Colour flow Doppler scan showing tibialis posterior tenosynovitis.

Plantar fascia

Inferior heel pain is a common clinical presentation and is usually due to plantar fasciitis. Inferior calcaneal bone spurs are common, but are not a cause of plantar fasciitis. Ultrasound is an objective method for confirming the diagnosis. The plantar fascia will become thickened, measuring more than 0.4 cm, with decreased reflectivity from oedema and thickening of the paratenon (*see* Figure 11.20). The paratenonitis is probably responsible for the pain, so it is logical to inject this area, rather than the tendon itself, which would run the risk of rupture. Ultrasound is an effective method for injecting the paratenon with steroid (which is difficult without image guidance as it is a very thin structure lying just superficial to the tendon) (*see* Figure 11.21).

The knee

MRI has an established role in, and is highly sensitive to, detecting meniscal and cruciate injury. Ultrasound is more limited, mainly because of the depth of structures. However, it is useful in diagnosing meniscal and parameniscal abnormality and is an effective tool in examining the patellar tendon. In some cases of patellar tendinosis there is cystic change, which is unlikely to settle with conservative management; therefore, appropriate orthopaedic referral should be considered.

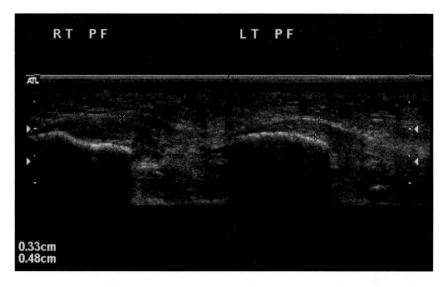

Figure 11.20 Plantar fasciitis demonstrating objective changes on ultrasound.

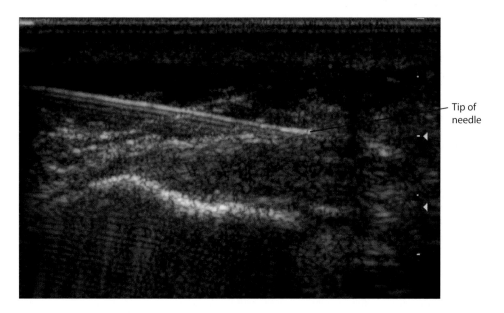

Figure 11.21 Ultrasound-guided injection of the paratenon around the plantar fascia.

ULTRASOUND IN INFLAMMATORY DISEASE

Ultrasound has been described as 'the rheumatologist's extended finger', emphasising its extended role in the clinical examination of musculoskeletal injury or disease. As there is no associated radiation, there is no limit to the number of examinations that can be performed. It has also been demonstrated to detect erosive changes earlier than conventional radiographs. Although proven to be as effective in this regard and capable of imaging areas that are inaccessible to ultrasound (e.g. the spine and sacroiliac joints), MRI is limited in terms of availability and cost.

The potential applications of ultrasound include:

- The examination of deep joints (i.e. the hip and shoulder).
- The detection of mild synovitis where clinical signs are absent.
- Distinction from synovitis and other causes of swelling, including tenosynovitis and subcutaneous oedema.
- Quantitative assessment of synovitis.
- Differentiation between synovial hypertrophy and effusion, allowing decisions regarding aspiration to be made.
- Needle placement for therapeutic injection, aspiration and biopsy.

Ultrasound-guided injection

Ultrasound-guided injection allows accurate injection into proven areas of abnormality. The needle tip is visible throughout the course of the examination, which allows a single and accurate passage into a bursa, small joint or paratenon. As the non-distended subacromial space measures less than 2 mm in width, accurate injection without guidance is difficult. Scanning during blind injections often shows the needle located within muscle or a tendon, with little resistance to injection.

The advantages of ultrasound-guided injection include quick and easy injection, the avoidance of multiple injections where there is lack of response and the certainty of accurate placement. There is little evidence to suggest that either a blind or guided injection confers any advantage, but this is the subject of current research.

Calcific tendinosis

Calcific tendinosis is a painful condition that can affect any tendon, although the supraspinatus tendon of the rotator cuff is the most commonly involved. The aetiology is unclear, although repetitive trauma, a genetic predisposition or biochemical disorder have all been implicated. Calcific deposits are common incidental findings and are thought to be painful during periods of formation and resorption. Patients often present with severe pain affecting all movements, which does not respond to local injection or anti-inflammatory drugs. While the diagnosis is commonly overlooked, once suspected, it can be confirmed with radiography or ultrasound. Ultrasound is useful in confirming that the pain is attributable

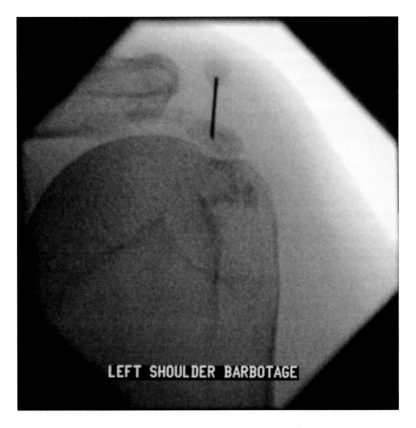

Figure 11.22 Calcific tendinosis: barbotage.

to the deposit and not impingement or a cuff tear. While the condition is often self-limiting, a significant number of patients will have a protracted course and further therapy should be considered.

Arthroscopic excision is a proven treatment, but it does carry all the attendant risks of surgery and anaesthesia, together with a long recovery period.

A percutaneous treatment is available (barbotage), which involves puncturing the deposit with two 20G needles inserted under ultrasound or fluoroscopic guidance. The procedure is performed under local anaesthesia and is well tolerated. Following multiple punctures, saline is washed through the deposit to remove some of the broken particles. Following the procedure, both steroid and Marcaine® are instilled before needle removal. The procedure takes about 15 minutes to perform and is sometimes followed by a 24-hour period of exacerbation of symptoms, with a marked improvement over the next few days. The procedure is thought to produce local hyperaemia, which aids resorption of the calcific deposits. Success has been reported in up to 90% of patients who have been recalcitrant to other methods of treatment, and where symptoms have lasted for many months (*see* Figure 11.22).

SHOCKWAVE THERAPY

Extracorporeal shockwave therapy (ESWT), previously known as extracorporeal shockwave lithotripsy (ESWL), has been available for some time and is a well-established and effective method for treating renal calculi. It also has an established role in treating bony and soft tissue disorders, with clinical improvement of symptoms in the following areas:

- Bony non-union.
- Calcific tendinosis.
- Tennis and golfer's elbow.
- Trochanteric bursitis.
- Patella tendinosis.
- Achilles tendinosis.
- Plantar fasciitis.
- Peyronie's disease of the penis.

ESWT directs shockwaves directly onto the affected tendon through ultrasound or radiographic guidance, and uses high-energy, accurately-focused beams of ultrasound waves. The mechanism of action is not entirely clear, but it can induce a local hyperaemic response, have an effect on cell membranes, alter the threshold of pain receptors or release negative ions, all of which are claimed to be responsible for its therapeutic response. ESWT is not widely available in the UK; there is greater experience of its use in the USA and mainland Europe. It has clear advantages in that it has no significant side effects, is non-invasive and does not involve the use of steroids. Results from those centres with wide experience of its use are encouraging and are the subject of ongoing research. Current European guidelines suggest its use in refractory tendinopathy, where there has been ineffective first-line therapy, including anti-inflammatory drugs, local steroid injection and physiotherapy.

EDUCATIONAL ASPECTS OF REPORTING

It will be difficult for practising clinicians to familiarise themselves with all the complex imaging and interventional techniques now available, but as requests are made and feedback is obtained, individual referrers will begin to develop a deeper understanding of the pathology and biomechanics of common soft tissue disorders. Through this process, clinicians will become more confident in their clinical management and recognise that there may be a reason why a problem has not improved with conservative management or injection. Imaging is also a useful tool for the practitioner, allowing prompt diagnosis and effective management, leading to patient and doctor satisfaction.

RESOURCE IMPLICATIONS

The availability of imaging modalities and therapeutic options varies geographically, so it is up to the clinical practitioner to make the most of what is available locally. Clinicians should develop a good relationship with providers in secondary care, who can then adapt their facilities to provide the best possible service to both patients and their doctors.

SUMMARY

Ultrasound and MRI can be used effectively to diagnose and treat a wide range of musculoskeletal conditions. The examples in this chapter are not exhaustive but have been chosen to illustrate the role of imaging and guided therapy in some of the more common soft tissue disorders. Imaging can be used to complement clinical diagnosis and injection techniques, allowing the practitioner to become more confident in his/her diagnosis and management of soft tissue disorders.

FURTHER READING

Blei CL *et al* (1986) Achilles tendon: ultrasound diagnosis of pathological conditions. *Radiology*. **159**: 765–767.

Bunker TD and Schranz PJ (1988) *Clinical Challenges in Orthopaedics: The Shoulder*. Oxford University Press, Oxford, UK.

Cunnane G *et al* (1996) Diagnosis and treatment of heel pain in chronic inflammatory arthritis using ultrasound. *Semin Arthritis Rheum*. **25**: 383–389.

Da Cruz DJ *et al* (1988) Achilles paratenonitis: An evaluation of steroid injection. *Br J Sports Med*. **22** (2): 64–65.

Farin PU and Jaroma H (1995) Acute traumatic tears of the rotator cuff: Value of sonography. *Radiology*. **197** (1): 269–273.

Farin PU *et al* (1995) Rotator cuff calcifications: treatment with US-guided technique. *Radiology*. **195**: 841–843.

Farin PU *et al* (1996) Rotator cuff calcifications: treatment with ultrasound-guided percutaneous needle aspiration and lavage. *Skeletal Radiol*. **25**: 551–554.

Gibbon WW *et al* (1999) Sonographic incidence of tendon microtears in athletes with chronic Achilles tendinosis. *Br J Sports Med*. **33** (2): 129–130.

Green S *et al* (2001) Interventions for shoulder pain. *Cochrane Database Syst Rev*. **2**: CD001156.

Hollister MS *et al* (1995) Association of sonographically detected subacromial/subdeltoid bursal effusion and intra-articular fluid with rotator cuff tear. *Am J Roentgenol*. **165**: 605–608.

Kane D *et al* (1998) Ultrasound guided injection of recalcitrant plantar fasciitis. *Ann Rheum Dis*. **57** (12): 749–750.

Loew M *et al* (1999) Shock-wave therapy is effective for chronic tendinosis of the shoulder. *J Bone Joint Surg Br*. **81** (5): 863–867.

Manger B and Kalden J (1995) Joint and connective tissue ultrasonography: a rheumatological bedside procedure? *Arthritis Rheum*. **38**: 736–742.

Rompe JD *et al* (1995) Extracorporal shock wave therapy for calcifying tendinitis of the shoulder. *Clin Orthop Relat Res.* **321**: 196–201.

Rompe JD *et al* (1998) Shoulder function after extracorporal shock wave therapy for calcific tendinitis. *J Shoulder Elbow Surg.* **7**: 505–509.

Index

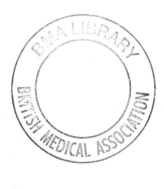